Advance Praise for THE PLANT ADVANTAGE

"The odds of losing a large amount of weight and keeping it off are small. Most people fail because they do not take an effective approach. For all those that say it can't be done, Benji Kurtz presents a proven plan that is both successful and health promoting." -Alan Goldhamer, Director of TrueNorth Health Center

"This book is a treasure. It is engaging, entertaining and enlightening. It is one of the rare "nutrition" books that is hard to put down. The story Benji Kurtz tells is one that millions of people can relate to. It is gives others hope for health. I wholeheartedly recommend reading it then sharing it with friends and family!" -Brenda Davis, RD, co-author of Becoming Vegan: Comprehensive and Express Editions

"Fueled by his own extraordinary journey, and fortified by relevant research, Benji offers us living proof that eating whole plant based foods is not only easy and accessible, but undeniably forms the diet of choice for us to achieve optimal human and environmental health. With refreshing wit and candor, The Plant Advantage is thoughtfully crafted to inspire us toward saving our life and along the way you will be saving the life of our planet." -Dr. Richard Oppenlander, Author of Comfortably Unaware and Food Choice and Sustainability, Executive Director of the non-profit Inspire Awareness Now, and lecturer and consultant

"Benji has synthesized all the pertinent scientific research on plant-based nutrition into one very enjoyable unique read. With his common sense approach and dry wit, he presents a very convincing path towards optimal health; for individuals, our country and for the planet. This is an entertaining, educational and practical book helping us understand why and how we should return to our natural herbivore roots!" -Neil Cooper MD, MHA, MSc Kaiser Permanente Workplace Wellness Team

The Plant Advantage

The Plant Advantage

HOW I LOST HALF MY WEIGHT ON THE
FUEL PLUS FORTIFICATION DIET

Benji Kurtz & Glen Merzer

ISBN-13: 9780692537008
ISBN-10: 0692537007
Library of Congress Control Number: 2015954824
Vivid Thoughts Press, Atlanta, GA

www.VividThoughtsPress.com

I suspect that the simple injunction "Do not eat animal products" has the potential to do more for world health than all of the abstruse wisdom in all of the world's medical libraries.

— Dr. Mark F. McCarty, biochemist who became vegan while researching the health effects of plant vs. animal proteins

Introduction

They call us "*homo sapiens.*" Actually, *we* call us "*homo sapiens.*" As conspiracy theorists need to learn, sometimes there is no "they." "*Homo,*" our genus, comes from the Latin, meaning "human being." "*Sapiens,*" our species, means "wise." And our subspecies, to which all modern humans belong, is called "*Homo sapiens sapiens,*" meaning, I think, "wise people who keep repeating the same dumb mistakes." In spite of those mistakes, we maintain a great deal of respect for ourselves, and so "*Homo*" is always capitalized.

But what sets us apart from other animals? What makes us unique (for surely we must be unique, or we wouldn't take so many selfies)? How are we different from the animals that we befriend and play with and teach tricks to and pamper as our pets, and the ones we gape at in awe on National Geographic specials, and the ones we breed and raise in captivity as our food?

For many years, it was believed that what makes humans human is our capacity to make tools; we were "man, the tool-maker." That was, until 1960, when Dr. Jane Goodall encountered a chimpanzee in Gombe Stream National Park in Tanzania that used grasses and twigs to catch insects. That single chimp did more than feast on termites; he undermined our pride as a species.

But that exasperating primate turned out not to be alone. Before we could nurse our resentment at him, we discovered that all kinds of other animals are also tool-makers, able to adapt objects in the environment to suit their purposes: to hunt for food, to create shelter, to groom themselves.

Orangutans use large leaves as umbrellas. Crows, like deranged avian stunt-men, actually use cars as tools: they drop nuts onto crosswalks to allow cars to run over them and break the shell, then they scoop up the shelled nuts when cars stop for red lights. (The crows' genius in using crosswalks compares favorably with the tactics of many pedestrians in the *Homo sapiens sapiens* camp.) Herons will use bread as a bait to catch fish. (But they cannot, as far as we know, bake the bread.) Bonobos make sponges from leaves for personal grooming. Dolphins use ready-made sea sponges as tools to forage for food on the sea floor. Elephants dig water holes with their tusks, then use chewed bark to plug them back up to prevent evaporation. They also employ branches for fly-swatting and back-scratching. Chimps crack nuts with stones. Vultures use stones to break eggs. Owls gather and deploy mammalian dung to attract dung beetles, which may be more delicious than we will ever know, unless we're lucky enough to be selected to appear in a reality show. Ants—lowly ants!—will form themselves into bridges so that their fellow ants can thereby walk over water, an example of intra-species cooperation clearly beyond the reach of *Homo sapiens*.

And so we can no longer define ourselves as "the toolmaker." Surely there must be some other crucial, innate characteristic that sets human animals apart from "pet" animals, "food" animals, and the glorious, untamed National Geographic animals?

I'm no taxonomist, but I believe I have the answer. We are, quite simply, the only animal that has no clue what to eat. This distinction applies, at least, to most of us living in the developed world, but I think it's fair to say that it applies to billions of us globally. I would humbly suggest we create a sub-subspecies that we call "*Homo sapiens sapiens perplexus.*" After all, you set every single other animal in the world out in the wild—every last one, mammal or bird or reptile or insect—and it knows exactly what to eat.

But, if you let a human being walk around in a grocery store, it gets agitated. *Should I get my milk low-fat or regular or should I flip the bird at the fat police and go for buttermilk? Are there too many carbs in these high-protein chips? Is this smelly cheese full of good fats or bad fats? How much sugar is in these colorful breakfast cereal thingies shaped like little hood ornaments? Is there gluten in Pringles, and what the hell is gluten, anyway? Is orange juice healthy, like the commercials say, or is it a carb? Is soy healthy, or is it a carcinogen? If pizza is bad for you, as everyone naturally agrees, is it because of the crust, the tomato sauce, the cheese, the mushrooms, or the pepperoni? Which is the best protein bar, and what did people do for protein before protein bars? What is the chemical used to add flavor to this fiber supplement, and why is it called "natural?" Is organic honey made from organic bees, and what makes a bee organic, anyway? Are these eggs free-range, and if so, did they roll around a lot in the grass? Is the skin safe to eat on a free-range chicken? For cooking, should I go with canola oil, olive oil, corn oil, safflower oil, coconut oil, butter, or a non-stick spray that says it's zero fat? What gives this salmon its bright orange glow, visible even in blackouts? Why do these cucumbers feel slicker than a greased pig? Is this scientifically formulated smoothie mix truly my ideal source of protein and calcium, like it says on the box? Is buffalo a lean meat, or does that depend on the buffalo?*

Homo sapiens sapiens perplexus. Members of the very same subspecies that boasts dominion over the earth. The masters of the universe. The ones who create art and culture. Who speak over six thousand distinct languages. Who have created ingenious ways for you to befriend countless people you will never meet or even speak with. Who can send a man to the moon, and never fail to remind themselves that since they did that, they should therefore be able to do a lot of other things that they never seem to be able to do. Humans, the nutritional idiots. The walking, talking animal so obtuse, it actually doesn't recognize its own food.

This book is meant to help you figure it out.

CHAPTER 1

Fat and Stupid

I hope this chapter title doesn't offend anyone. I'm not saying that fat people are stupid. I'm saying that I was fat, and I was stupid.

I was overweight most of my life. I was certainly plump by the time I was ten, if not sooner than that. It wasn't like I was raised in a family that just wasn't paying attention. My mother was careful to serve me *lean meats* and a *balanced diet*. I didn't eat candy and I didn't ingest soda. I never had an eating disorder; I never binged or purged. My parents were both of normal weight, although I was familiar with the story that my father had lost about sixty pounds early in my parents' marriage, before I was born. I had seen the pictures of him at about 230 pounds, in which he was unrecognizable. That knowledge served always as my clue that there was a bad gene for weight gain in the family, and I assumed that— my bad luck—it had worked its way into my chromosomes. *Thanks a lot, Dad*, I thought.

I am five-foot-five inches tall, and slight of build. So, I had no business reaching the weight of 180 or so that I achieved in high school. At that point, I was a good forty pounds overweight, on the borderline of obesity. I certainly indulged a little too often in the chips or other snacks I was able to obtain from the school's vending machines, but the bulk of my calories were consumed at home, where I dutifully ingested the "healthy, balanced" meals my mother prepared for the family, and so those carefully thought-out meals clearly must have been the major contributors to my weight gain. Still, I was closer to a normal weight in high school than in college. As soon as I left my home town of Athens, Georgia, to live independently at Emory University in Atlanta, I took advantage of my newfound freedom to indulge in a lot of pizza, *Chick-Fil-A*, and a general Food Court eating style. There were a lot of late nights at *Waffle House*, and plenty of burgers or cheeseburgers and fries. Perhaps not surprisingly, during what should have been my physically active college days (but were instead my sedentary college days), I ballooned up to 250 pounds. I became not just obese, but morbidly obese.

If you had asked me at that time why I thought I had become more than a hundred pounds overweight—a subject I tried not to think about too much—I would probably have said that it was a combination of lack of exercise, eating too many high-carb comfort foods, and my Dad's evil gene.

For the next 18 years, I became the poster child for the yo-yo dieter. I tried all manner of diets: *Jenny Craig, Weight Watchers*, the *South Beach Diet*, the *Atkins Diet, Slimfast* shakes, and my own tweaks and hybrids of all of the above. I learned a crucial lesson about diet plans: they all work. Really. I lost considerable weight each time I went on every last one of those diets. As long as you stick to the protocol, you really will lose weight. All these diets revolved around one or two basic concepts: calorie restriction, and/or depriving the body of sufficient carbohydrate so that it will instead burn fat and protein, putting the body into a dangerous state called ketosis, and causing temporary water-weight loss that jump-starts the diet.

So I was a very successful dieter, every time, usually for a few months at a time. I would lose thirty or forty pounds, for as long as I could stand to be on the diet, and then I'd gain it all back, and then some, in short order after I grew tired of the restrictions and after my body cried out for some carbohydrate.

I'm sure you've met a smoker who says, "I can quit any time. I've already quit twenty-five times, so it's absolutely no problem." I was that kind of dieter. Like so many millions of Americans, I found that the challenge wasn't taking the weight off; the challenge was keeping the weight off. The diets ceased to work once the calorie restriction became unbearable, and once my body cried out for foods, like pasta, that I wasn't permitted.

Besides, some of the meal plans just weren't feasible. *Jenny Craig* involved a system of having frozen meals sent to me, and eating only those meals. Where on earth was I supposed to keep frozen meals while living in a college dorm and working thirty hours a week at a radio station? *Weight Watchers* also offered frozen meals, along with a regimen of group meetings that were heavy on inspiration. It was hard to tolerate. I didn't need to be inspired; I needed to lose weight and keep it off. I was a young guy trying to get on with my life, and every minute spent listening to a group of overweight *yentas* cheer each other on for dropping three pounds was a minute I knew I would never get back. I found those inspirational sessions profoundly dispiriting.

In the years 2003 and 2004, I was provided with a legitimate, extra dose of inspiration: I got engaged to my high school sweetheart, Claire. I never worked harder to lose weight. For six months, I restricted my calories, avoided the dreaded "carbs" that everybody knew caused weight gain, followed the protocol of my own blend of the South Beach and Atkins diets, worked out in the gym, lifted weights, and walked at least three miles a day. By our wedding day I had lost thirty pounds and was down to 204. And then on our honeymoon, in Paris and the Maldives, I stuffed myself, and gained ten pounds.

My weight continued to yo-yo after that, but generally each high point of the oscillation was higher than the last. I kept setting new personal records for morbid obesity. The heaviest point that I recorded on a scale was 278, but likely I went higher, since I was loathe to step on a scale while I was in that range; I would sometimes stop weighing myself for months at a time. None of my successful diets ever brought me below my not-so-svelte wedding weight of 204.

And remember, I never ate junk food, never drank alcohol or soda pop, never binged on sweets. I am not now, and never have been, a food addict. I never gorged on whole gallons of ice cream, or even pints. If I wanted dessert, a couple of spoonfuls of ice cream would satisfy me. For the most part, I simply ate normal, healthy, "balanced" meals, like chicken and broccoli cooked in olive oil and butter. Grilled salmon with green beans on the side. A little "lean" protein, some vegetables, a nice sauce. I wasn't above indulging in some American comfort food classics: the occasional pizza or spaghetti with meat balls or mac'n'cheese or cheeseburgers. In fact, during my South Beach or Atkins diets, I would have the cheeseburger without the bun. In a lettuce wrap, a cheeseburger was an ideal, healthy meal. Meat, cheese, condiments—and with it all wrapped up in lettuce without any dreaded "carbs," what could be healthier? I didn't eat great quantities of anything; I ate normal, sensible portions. I never boasted an enormous appetite, although I managed to achieve an enormous weight without it. The pounds attached themselves to me like paparazzi to a Kardashian. It was that damned gene from my father.

My mind came to associate weight loss with struggle, restriction, and heroic effort; weight gain, by contrast, was simply the natural result of eating normal-sized meals when I was hungry and not forcing myself to exercise strenuously.

I did not particularly want to see people socially because I did not want to be seen. It's no way to go through life, hoping to stay away from social events as much as possible, but that was how I lived.

Obesity became a central fact of my life, if one that was rarely discussed. I didn't feel good about myself. I felt shame without guilt; I had done nothing wrong, yet had become a person unworthy, in my own eyes, of society. I detested going shopping for clothes, something that could successfully be accomplished only at the Big and Tall shops. Even then, it was a nuisance to search for the only items that might fit me, all the way to the right of the rack. There aren't too many good choices at size 50. At that size, the only thing that's slim is the pickings. It was also humiliating to ask for the seat belt extender on airplanes, or to have to sit on special vehicles on amusement park rides. When I drove, my car seat had to be far back enough to accommodate my gut, but close enough for my feet to reach the pedals; this became more and more tricky as I packed on the pounds. Although I liked to swim as a child (and I like to swim again now), I didn't go in a pool from the age of ten until the age of thirty-seven because I was mortified at the prospect of taking my shirt off and exposing my fat in front of others. It simply was not fun to be viewed at all. I knew people were thinking about how overweight I was, even though nobody ever said anything about it. I wasn't interested in a social existence, and that lack of desire to be around people took its toll on my personality, and inevitably on my happiness.

My size colored my relationships with everyone, including my loving parents. I can certainly appreciate the tough spot they were in. They didn't want to harp on my weight as I was growing up, and make me feel unloved or unappreciated, but at the same time, given that they had my best interests at heart, how could they ignore my consistent weight gain? So from time to time they would express their disapproval without harping on the subject. I didn't take it well. I never appreciated being criticized. It wasn't news to me that I was fat. It was embarrassing to talk about, even with my parents. These talks tapered off as I became an adult; they knew they were no longer responsible for my well-being. But I knew what they were thinking even when they weren't expressing their thoughts.

Perhaps my interest in radio would have developed even had my size been normal, but certainly a career in radio seemed the perfect choice for someone like me who was trying not to be seen. In radio, I could work in a windowless room and even get some attention without anyone knowing what I looked like. As a thirteen-year-old kid, I read the news and even was given an editorial slot—*The Kurtz Korner*—on a local talk station, *WBKZ*. (Perhaps you recall my scathing editorial broadside against the chess club budget cuts?) I would go on to become a radio jack-of-all-trades: disc jockey, public service director, board operator, program director, group operations manager, producer, consultant. My career in radio helped me survive, but, given my obesity, a kind of low-key, insulated, reclusive survival was the best I could hope for.

I never admitted to myself that my weight was out of my control. I told myself I would get it under control someday, with a prolonged period of eating nothing but meat and fruits and vegetables and no "carbs." At some point, I assured myself, I would get around to doing that, not just for a few months, as I had so many times before, but for however long it took, probably years.

It was obvious that I would never be thin. My goal was more realistic. I was shooting for chunky. To go from morbidly obese to chunky would represent an extraordinary achievement, and I could live with being chunky. Hell, I would have even been proud of attaining a merely chunky physique. But that goal, modest as it might sound, seemed to recede from possibility year after year. Chunky was just a dream I had.

Stupidly, it never occurred to me, over twenty-five years of failed weight-loss attempts, to question all the nutritional assumptions that had been drilled into me. It never occurred to me to ask whether it was possible that the best-selling diet books and weight-loss programs—which, after all, I knew worked very well, at least to help me lose an initial twenty or thirty pounds—could all be completely off the mark, and designed simply to fool the public and to make their authors wealthy as they made their readers unhealthy, and ultimately kept them fat. It never occurred to me to ask whether the type of food I'd been eating all my life might not be sensible or appropriate for humans to eat at all.

It never occurred to me to ask, in effect, what is my body designed to eat?

And then, one night at home, I saw a movie, and it changed my life.

More about that movie and my weight-loss later, but first, let's take the time to answer the question that I was foolish enough to not ask myself during an agonizing, quarter-century-long struggle with obesity: what is human food?

CHAPTER 2

Human Food

I f I tell you that sharks are designed to eat fish, I'm sure you'll agree. If I tell you that lions and tigers are designed to eat large mammals, you will have no quarrel. Owls are masterful predators designed to eat small mammals like rodents, insects, and, terrifyingly enough, their fellow birds. Horses, elephants, cows, and giraffes, despite their massive size and strength, are some of nature's gentlest creatures—not predators, but vegetarians, as we all know. (The human experiment with feeding cows the tissue of other cows turned out not to work out so well, leading to Mad Cow Disease, yet the experiment continues in another form as cows are still fed other animal remains in the form of roadkill and euthanized pets and chicken droppings and cow blood.)

But what is a human? A natural predator and omnivore or a natural herbivore (plant-eater)?

One answer to that question is given by the fad diet of the day, the Paleo Diet, founded by Dr. Loren Cordain, who has his own meat-heavy dietary prescriptions like those of the late Dr. Robert Atkins, who, like Cordain, was himself fat. The central thesis of the Paleo Diet is that humans should eat as our Paleolithic ancestors evolved to eat before the dawn of agriculture 10,000 years ago. We therefore should eat a diet,

Cordain claims, that is roughly 19-35% protein, emphasizing protein from animal foods and especially grass-fed animal foods, since cavemen didn't have Concentrated Animal Feeding Operations (CAFOs). The diet excludes grains, viewed as the unnatural and unhealthy product of the perverse modern practice known as agriculture, and instead promotes the foods that humans allegedly evolved to eat before heading down the dark, dangerous, Faustian path of cultivating plants. The whole premise of the diet is torn to shreds in a delightful Ted Talk given by Christina Warinner [1], Ph.D., director of the Laboratories of Molecular Anthropology and Microbiome Research (LMAMR) and an Assistant Professor of Anthropology at the University of Oklahoma. Unlike Cordain, Warriner, an archeological scientist, speaks with professional expertise when she points out that her research on the teeth of ancient humans leads to the conclusion that there was an "abundance of plant remains inside the dental calculus of Paleolithic peoples ... including grains ... legumes and tubers." [2]

Remember: grains, legumes, and tubers (starchy vegetables) are no-no's on the Paleo Diet, precisely because our ancestors did not eat them. Or at least they weren't supposed to. They were supposed to be busy hunting and creating the first barbecues in caves, and serving up their burgers without buns. So if in fact they were eating a lot of berries and grains and starchy vegetables, that's a very inconvenient fact for the Paleo industry.

How then does the Paleo camp spin the revelation that Paleolithic people in fact ate grain and starchy vegetables? Here's what Robb Wolf, an acolyte of Cordain and author of "The Paleo Solution," has to say: "As to the grain/legume consumption itself, it still begs the questions of what is really healthy to eat, particularly as a preponderance of calories" [3]

I find this pretty hilarious. First, the Paleo advocates say we should eat the way the "caveman" ate because that's the way humans are meant to eat; then, when it turns out that the "caveman" in fact ate plant foods that are prohibited in the Paleo diet, they say, in effect, "Well, what difference does *that* make? It doesn't prove that it's healthy."

Indeed. Point taken. The fact that "cavemen" did or did not eat something doesn't prove that it's the optimal diet. In Paleolithic times, the human lifespan, usually estimated at no more than thirty-five [4], was a fraction of what it is today. The goal today is to live a long life, even a hundred years or more, in optimal health. In Paleolithic times, the imperative was simply to live long enough to procreate. That's why 401(k) plans were not available in Paleolithic times; lengthy retirements were uncommon. The goal was to reproduce before you could be killed by, say, a scratch.

The Paleo Diet does accommodate non-starchy vegetables like lettuce, broccoli, and Brussels sprouts, but as Warriner points out, these foods are actually the result of the newfangled, Paleo-maligned practice known as agriculture: the lettuce and broccoli and Brussels sprouts that we eat today, and that the Paleo Diet approves of, did not exist before agriculture; humans have domesticated these plants to make them more tasty and in some cases more caloric. So if we should only eat foods that existed in the form that the "caveman" encountered them, virtually all fruits and vegetables that you find in the produce aisle of your grocery store should be *verboten*.

I like to think civilization has progressed at least a trifle since Paleolithic times, which ended ten thousand years ago. Science has advanced more than a little bit since the discovery of fire. Is there any reason under the stars that instead of turning to science to help us determine what is most healthy for our bodies, we should instead try to guess what our ancestors ate while they lived in an environment vastly different from our own, with food choices vastly different than our own, and then attempt to eat the way we imagine they did? It's a pretty insane way to construct and justify a dietary program, but it has managed to sell a lot of books.

So let's start with an understanding, which I'm guessing our cave-dwelling ancestors did not have, of the macronutrient composition of foods. Flesh foods tend to provide just less than one-half of their calories as protein and just more than one-half as fat. They have no carbohydrate and no fiber. Eating a diet consisting of flesh foods only would be unthinkable. A person trying it would become severely malnourished. The Inuit (with a not terribly enviable life expectancy in the mid-sixties), [5] eat a diet that leans about as heavily on flesh foods as any human population, and their bones suffer the consequences. "Aging bone loss, which occurs in many populations, has an earlier onset and greater intensity in the Eskimos. Nutrition factors of high protein, high nitrogen, high phosphorus, and low calcium intakes may be implicated." [6] Still, even the Inuit eat tubers, berries, seaweed, and other plants, and they rely on the environmental advantage that the blubber of raw or frozen marine mammals contain glycogen stores that serve as a source of carbohydrate. That is an advantage virtually all Americans do not have when they eat a meat-heavy diet. Morgan Spurlock's documentary "Supersize Me" gives a vivid demonstration of what happens to the average person's weight and health when he limits himself to a fatty diet composed mainly of flesh foods and dairy, topped off with oily French fries and Coke; it's remarkable how quickly his health deteriorates from three McDonald's meals a day, endangering his life within a month.

By contrast, eating a diet with absolutely no animal foods is perfectly achievable, and is easily accomplished by millions of people around the world, usually to the benefit of their health.

Of the three macronutrients, carbohydrate is the one burned most cleanly by the human body for energy. And the brain runs on glucose, the simplest form of carbohydrate. Carbohydrate is a molecule composed of carbon, the stuff of life, and water, the stuff of life. How exactly did a molecule that basic to human existence develop such a bad reputation?

So when we compare the macronutrient compositions of flesh foods and plant foods, we have to begin with the fact that flesh foods lack carbohydrate, the optimal human fuel. You can't live without carbohydrate.

Advantage: plants.

Next, we turn to fat. If you ever forget which of the three macronutrients contribute the most to weight gain, there is a subtle clue in the word "fat." Most flesh foods are more than 50% fat, and much of that is saturated fat, a contributor to heart disease. As the American diet has increased in the absolute intake of fat (although the *percentage* of calories from fat in the diet may have decreased slightly because of an even greater caloric increase in sugar), obesity has skyrocketed. With more than twice as many calories in a gram of fat as in a gram of carbohydrate or protein, it shouldn't come as a surprise that fat makes you fat.

Medical professionals and dietitians disagree about the optimal percentage of calories as fat in the diet, and it will vary with the age, weight, physical activity and genetic profile of the individual, but it's probably safe to say that you want to be in the range of 10-20% of calories as fat, and surely not at 30% or above. (The average American consumes about 35% of calories in the form of fat.) Fat in the bloodstream can inhibit insulin receptors in the cells from doing their job of metabolizing glucose, and that can lead to type 2 diabetes. This is not new information; it has been established for some time. A 1935 study of fat vs. carbohydrate consumption in various cultures showed that as carbohydrate intake increases and fat intake decreases, mortality associated with diabetes plummets by about 86%. [7] Somehow, that evidence that has been with us for eighty years has not been sufficient to motivate most medical professionals and governmental bureaucrats in the dietary guideline business to question the wildly high percentage of fat in the typical American diet. While some plant foods are fatty—nuts, seeds, avocados, olives, and coconut, for example—most fruits, vegetables, legumes and grains are low in fat, and constructing a diet around those foods is the only way you can healthfully get into that 10-20% range.

Advantage: plants.

Ah, but what about protein? For years, we were taught that the superior protein is found in animal foods. On restaurant menus around the country, the euphemism for flesh foods has become "protein." (How often have you seen, *"Choice of protein: beef, fish, chicken."* I have yet to run across a menu that says, *"Choice of saturated fat and cholesterol: beef, fish, chicken."* Protein is more highly regarded than saturated fat and cholesterol, so it has become synonymous with flesh foods.) Everything we have traditionally been taught about the superiority of animal protein turns out to be untrue. In point of fact, plant protein is eminently superior to animal protein. In their groundbreaking work, *The China Study*, T. Colin Campbell and Thomas Campbell explain that high-protein diets are carcinogenic, particularly if the protein is animal-derived. As the Campbells concluded from the most comprehensive study of nutrition ever undertaken, "nutrients from animal-based foods increased tumor development while nutrients from plant-based foods decreased tumor development." [8] This was particularly the case with proteins. Animal protein is also more sulfuric and acidic than plant protein, and as a consequence has been implicated in osteoporosis. Methionine, the sulfuric amino acid more abundant in animal than plant protein, also has been associated with tumor stimulation.

Advantage: plants.

Fiber is indispensable in the human diet, and is sometimes referred to as the fourth macronutrient. A diet high in fiber will contribute to weight loss by helping us feel satiated. Fiber also regulates the absorption of sugar into the bloodstream, thereby reducing the risk of type 2 diabetes. Fiber has also been shown to lower serum cholesterol levels. And, of course, fiber keeps the bowels in good working order. Fiber is found only in plants.

Advantage: plants.

Okay, we're done with the macronutrients, but what about the micronutrients? After all, everyone agrees on the importance of having antioxidants in your diet to ward off cancer.

Antioxidants are found only in plants.

Advantage: plants.

Folate, a nutrient that is known for its role in preventing fetal deformities, and that also helps ward off cancer and Alzheimer's, is most readily available in dark leafy greens and legumes. The richest sources of Vitamin C are citrus fruits and any number of vegetables, such as red peppers. Those are but two examples of micronutrients most easily obtained by eating plant foods, but of course plant foods are part of an omnivorous diet. In truth, most vitamins and minerals can be obtained sufficiently from both plant and animal sources. In most cases, the animals obtained those micronutrients in the first place by eating plants. The single micronutrient for which there is an inherent advantage in animal foods is Vitamin B-12. On a diet that contains no animal foods (a vegan diet), taking a B-12 supplement once or twice a week is strongly recommended. (B-12 can also be obtained by eating fortified foods.) So, when it comes to vitamins and minerals, there's no particular advantage in obtaining all you need with either a strictly herbivorous diet (as long as you supplement with B-12) or an omnivorous diet.

Let's return now to the question of whether humans are designed to be herbivores or omnivores. We have seen that the macronutrient profile of plant foods is more conducive to human health than the macronutrient profile of animal products, and that fiber and antioxidants, only available in plant foods, are crucial components of a healthful diet. But omnivores could argue that, since plant foods are welcome in their diet, they could still get plenty of fiber and antioxidants. Still, they would have to concede that, on a per-calorie basis, they'd be getting less fiber and less antioxidant power on the omnivorous diet than on a whole-foods, plant-based diet. In other words, if we're going to compare a 2,000 calorie diet composed only of whole, plants foods with a 2,000 calorie diet in which 500 calories come from flesh foods and another 500 calories come from dairy (and the rest from whole, plant foods), you could expect to have roughly half as much fiber and half as much antioxidant power on the omnivorous diet. And with less fiber, you might expect less of a feeling of satiation with your 2,000 calories, so that could easily cause you to increase your intake to 2,200 or 2500 calories on the omnivorous diet to feel as full. Those extra calories would of course lead to weight gain. An extra 500 calories per day could lead to an extra pound added to your frame weekly.

Blood pressure is a fundamental and simple gauge of health, so what have we learned about blood pressure on a herbivorous vs. an omnivorous diet? In 2002, a significant British study analyzed the risk of hypertension in more than 2,000 males and nearly 9,000 female participants, divided between meat eaters, fish eaters, vegetarians, and vegans. Vegans were least likely to report hypertension (5.8% of men and 7.7% of women); meat eaters were most likely (15% of men and 12.1% of women). Hypertension in fish eaters and vegetarians was between that of meat-eaters and vegans. Similarly, meat eaters had the highest measured blood pressure; vegans had the lowest values; fish eaters and vegetarians had similar values that were in-between. Non-meat eaters, especially vegans, were the leanest. Vegans had the lowest risk of heart disease and stroke due to lower blood pressure. [9]

A 1996 study of more than 50,000 male health professionals demonstrated that those who ate the most fiber had a reduced risk of coronary heart disease. [10] Now, is this because the fiber itself, perhaps by lowering serum cholesterol levels, prevented heart disease? Or could it be because those who ate the most fiber presumably ate the least non-fibrous foods—flesh foods and dairy—and therefore ate the least saturated fat? Or could it be because of heart-healthy attributes in vegetables and fruit, like antioxidants, that were enjoyed in greater measure by those on the higher fiber diet? Most likely, we will never know. But we don't have to be able to answer these questions to detect a pattern in the nutritional evidence that points us in the direction of knowing what constitutes a healthy diet. It seems that there are countless health attributes to plant-based foods—science is always discovering more—and countless risks involved in consuming flesh foods and the lactation of other species.

Another study, this one of over 25,000 Seventh-Day Adventists in California, found that daily meat-eaters had a three times greater likelihood of dying from heart disease than those who did not eat meat. [11]

Virtually all studies you will find lead to the same conclusion: plant foods confer a myriad of health benefits that researchers continue to discover; animal foods lead to inflammation, unhealthy levels of cholesterol, weight gain, higher blood pressure, heart disease, higher risk of various cancers, and higher incidence of all-cause mortality. Yes, it's true that studies that confer some benefits to fatty fish have been ballyhooed; it has been shown that consuming fatty fish like salmon and mackerel lead to reduced risk of sudden cardiac death. But these studies are always comparing fish-eaters to meat-eaters, not to those on a low-fat, plant-based diet. So, the best news about any animal-based food may be that eating sea animals may be less harmful to your health than eating land animals. And even that is debatable.

We have seen that an understanding of the macronutrient profile of plant and animal foods gives us good reason to doubt that there is any role for animal foods in the human diet. We have also seen that nutritional research adds more weight to the conclusion that humans are natural herbivores. But all the same, weren't we designed to be caveman hunters, as the Paleo Diet peddlers would have us believe?

Again, the fact that our ancestors who inhabited caves engaged in hunting (while also consuming all manner of plant food) tells us nothing about what the optimal human diet should be. Those primitive hunters just needed sufficient calories to survive long enough to reproduce; they weren't particularly worried about developing heart disease in their sixties or seventies.

No tenable case can be made that humans were in any way designed by nature to eat meat; the science of comparative anatomy makes this remarkably clear. We have simply none of the physical characteristics of carnivores and omnivores that make flesh an appropriate food for them.

Dr. Milton Mills, a practicing physician in Virginia and the Associate Director of Preventive Medicine with the Physician's Committee for Responsible Medicine, makes perhaps the most clear and definitive analysis of the diet we humans were designed to eat in his essay, "The Comparative Anatomy of Eating." [12] It would be well worth anyone's time to read that short essay, but let me summarize its main points here.

Like all other mammalian herbivores, Dr. Mills points out, humans do not have the wide mouth opening that carnivores make use of to kill other animals. Like all other mammalian herbivores, our jaws and facial muscles are not designed for tearing apart flesh, but rather for grinding. Like all other mammalian herbivores, we chew our food; carnivores and omnivores swallow it whole. Like all other mammalian herbivores, we have starch-digesting enzymes in our saliva; carnivores and omnivores do not. Like all other mammalian herbivores, we have weak stomach acid, demonstrating a pH in the range of 4-5 with food in our stomachs; carnivores and omnivores have strong stomach acid to support the digestion of meat, boasting a pH of 1 or less with food in their stomachs. Our stomach capacity in relation to the volume of our digestive tract is less than half of that of carnivores or omnivores, and similar to that of other mammalian herbivores. Like all other mammalian herbivores, our small intestines are at least ten times our body length, as opposed to three to six times body length for carnivores and four to six times body length for omnivores. Like all other mammalian herbivores, we do not have the highly concentrated urine of carnivores or omnivores. Like all other mammalian herbivores, we do not have the claws that all carnivores and omnivores employ for predation; instead, we have hands that serve us well in picking fruit and, dare I mention it, agriculture.

Wouldn't it seem that these facts alone should put to bed the question of whether humans are natural herbivores, rather than omnivores? Alas, facts and logic can always be countered by committed ideologues, and so the Paleo-friendly website www.beyondveg.com makes this argument to counter the obvious truths brought to light by Dr. Mills: "*Technology, driven by our intelligence, supports adaptive behavior that allows us to easily overcome the physical limitations that the comparative 'proofs' regard (incorrectly) as being limiting factors. Along similar lines, we don't need the strong bodies of a lion or tiger because we have something much more powerful: high intelligence, which allowed humans to become the most efficient hunters, and the dominant mammalian species, on the planet.*" [13]

If you ponder this argument for a moment, it will take your breath away. Here's a diet—an entire industry, really—premised on the seemingly reasonable idea that evolution is destiny, that we should endeavor to eat today the same kind of foods that we ate tens of thousands of years ago. Humans are natural meat-eaters, claim the Paleo enthusiasts, because we evolved to eat meat as hunters before the unnatural invention of agriculture ten thousand years ago. Ten thousand years has not been long enough, they say, for our bodies to adjust to such unnatural foods as wheat, barley, corn and rice, which, they claim, are making us fat and sick.

Then, when faced with overwhelming evidence that every last characteristic of our digestive system and our physiology, aspects of our inherent physical nature that evolved over literally *millions* of years, places us squarely in the camp of herbivores, just like our primate cousins, the meat enthusiasts respond, in effect, by saying, "Well, evolution doesn't matter in the case of humans because we are so smart that we have overcome our physical limitations by inventing stun guns and electric prods, meat hooks, knives, and charcoal grills, so now it's perfectly healthy, and indeed required, for us to eat meat."

Because we can.

Yes, we can, but it's clearly the animal products in our diet that are making us fat and sick, not the wheat, barley, corn, and rice, and one has to be willfully blind not to see it. That's precisely why so many people in Asian societies who have moved away from a traditional diet based on rice towards a rich Western diet based on animal products have begun to fall victim to diabetes, obesity, heart disease, and cancer.

I lost half my body weight, and all my health metrics improved dramatically, in the year-and-a-half when I first moved away from a diet centered on animal products to a diet centered on the very foods that the Paleo enthusiasts warn us about. I have since met many others with similar stories. How do the Paleo enthusiasts explain us?

They can't, of course, but as a last rhetorical refuge they may ask in turn: *if humans weren't designed to be meat-eaters, why do we have a taste for the flesh of other animals?*

Here's my best guess, and it's an informed guess that I make on the basis of my extraordinary expertise as a guy who used to be extremely fat. Meat is fatty. Fat is calorie-dense. When the principle challenge for our ancestors was to obtain enough calories to survive, nature effectively put a premium on fatty foods. And so, as a species, we have a weakness for the taste of something that isn't designed to be our natural food. Does anyone argue that ice cream is a healthy food? But humans clearly have a taste for that as well. In the case of ice cream, it's both the fat and the sugar that humans crave. We also have a taste for salted peanuts and for potato chips and corn chips and for chocolate cake with frosting and sprinkles. The fact that we exhibit a "taste" for something doesn't mean that we should eat it.

True carnivores and omnivores don't merely exhibit a "taste" for animal foods; they exhibit an instinct to kill and eat them raw. Do you have any desire, when you see a chicken, to bite its head off? Any desire to bite into the living flesh of a cow, a pig, a deer, a rabbit?

As a general rule, we eat our meat disguised, cooked and covered in sauces, precisely because we have no instinct for predation.

Carnivorous animals can eat essentially unlimited amounts of fat without developing atherosclerosis; that's certainly not true of humans.

But are there any essential nutrients that people obtain from flesh foods and dairy that can't be easily obtained on an herbivorous diet?

Except for Vitamin B-12, the answer is no. There's no problem obtaining enough protein or iron or calcium or any other nutrient that you may have heard is deficient on a plant-based diet. It's simply not the case. When you hear that dairy products are essential for calcium, ask yourself where the cows got the calcium in the first place—and the answer is, obviously, from eating plant foods. Calcium is a mineral in the ground that is absorbed into growing plants, such as grass; that's where the dietary calcium cycle starts, not in the teats of cows. Children raised on a vegan diet who never eat a bite of meat or have a glass of cow milk or a piece of traditional cheese (as opposed to plant-based cheeses) nonetheless thrive.

Obtaining Vitamin B-12 on a vegan diet might not be so difficult if we didn't engage in the sensible practice of washing our vegetables, as it is found in the bacteria in the soil. A Vitamin B-12 deficiency can lead to such serious conditions as pernicious anemia. While the original source of B-12 is bacteria, omnivorous and carnivorous species can obtain it by eating animals. On a vegan diet, it can be obtained through fortified foods and fermented foods, but a B-12 supplement is recommended, just to be safe, by all responsible advocates of a plant-based diet.

So, you may ask, can it really be true that humans have absolutely no need for animal foods, that animal foods are, in fact, detrimental to human health, while the overwhelming majority of people around the world continue to eat them? How can that possibly be? Am I saying that people are simply foolish?

That's a tough question to answer. Some of my best friends are people, so I'm not going to level any accusations. But yes, as a nation and as a world we are engaged in a kind of collective insanity. We are constructing our diets around substances that are not our natural human food, and we're destroying our planet in the process. We have arrived at this point for many reasons:

1. Humans have a weakness for fatty foods in general;
2. Our ancestors ate meat because obtaining sufficient caloric intake was their primary goal, not longevity;
3. It is only recently that large-scale animal agriculture has posed a threat to the planet;
4. Eating animals became associated in many cultures with strength and power;
5. Science initially made the error of attributing superiority to animal protein;
6. Culture and habit die hard, and eating animals is common in most cultures;
7. The human body is durable and pliant, and so there are many long-lived meat-eaters, who appear to provide evidence against the truth that animal foods are unnecessary and harmful;
8. Nutritional studies are designed and presented in ways that appear confusing and contradictory to the general public, and rarely involve a cohort on low-fat, plant-based diets;
9. The industry of animal agriculture promotes its interests without compunction, taking good advantage of a confused public, and infiltrating all agencies of government relevant to advancing sales of their products;

10. It isn't only animal foods that are making Americans fat and sick; it is also excessive ingestion of certain types of plant foods, most notably oils and sugars and white flour. This provides ammunition to the defenders of the meat industry who can point these substances as the true evils in our diet, and to the less-than-stellar health outcomes of an unfortunate subset of plant-based eaters on poor diets.

For all these reasons and more, what should be obvious by now to all—that human beings are natural herbivores who do a disservice to their health with every bite of animal food—remains obscure to most.

As long as Americans are confused about nutrition, we will continue to be fat and sick. We need to have an understanding of the basic principles involved in human nutrition. That begins with an understanding that the way we eat will affect our health more than virtually anything else.

CHAPTER 3

Fuel Plus Fortification

et me suggest a way to think about nutrition and the decisions we make every day about what to eat: your nutritional goal should be *fuel plus fortification*. Of course, eating is also a source of pleasure, but that isn't the subject of the body of this book (though it's a leading consideration of the recipe section).

Let's say you're really hungry, having worked hard doing some kind of physical labor all day, and now you feel the need to have a big dinner to satisfy your hunger and renew your energy stores. But the only food to be found is in a cafeteria, where you are offered three options: 1) a large raw salad of lettuce, tomato, cucumber, radishes, celery, and alfalfa sprouts; 2) a large meatloaf, with a side of steamed broccoli; 3) a large burrito made of rice and beans.

Now remember: you're really hungry. All three meals fill up a good-sized plate. Which would you, or should you, choose?

That salad sounds awfully healthy. Raw vegetables full of live enzymes and antioxidants, and every ounce of it full of fiber. There's absolutely nothing but vibrant health to that salad. But you know you're still going to be hungry after you eat it. It will not be a satisfying meal.

The salad gets points for being healthy, but it doesn't get many points as fuel. There might be only 100 calories to that whole, big salad. (Though you could add hundreds more by soaking it in an unhealthy, oily dressing.) You've been working hard all day; you need some calories, and a full feeling in your stomach.

The meatloaf will fill you up all right. It has over 600 calories. It also has some 40 grams of fat, 15 grams of saturated fat, and 110 milligrams of cholesterol. Its percentage of calories as fat is around 60%. So, while it will fill you up, it'll also speed you along towards heart disease, contributing more saturated fat in one meal than you should have in at least a week. Its high fat content will make your blood fatty, potentially interfering with the insulin receptors in your cells and contributing to diabetes. As fuel, meatloaf is undesirable because it has no carbohydrate; if you were to rely on it alone for fuel, you would need to burn either its fat or its protein—both processes that stress the body and throw off toxic byproducts. It has no fiber. In short, meatloaf is not human food and it will contribute to weight gain and have a pernicious effect on your health. And while that side of steamed broccoli is terrific, it can't begin to undo the harm of the meatloaf.

The correct answer, of course, is the bean-and-rice burrito. It will have about 250 calories, 9 grams of protein, 44 grams of carbohydrate, and only a few grams of fat (as it hopefully will be prepared without oil). Its percentage of calories as fat should be in the 10-15% range. It will have 6 grams of fiber and will fill you up; if it doesn't, then be my guest, have two burritos.

Okay, one more quiz. It's time for breakfast. You have a big day ahead of you, and you want to start the day with an optimally nutritious meal. Should you start the day with: 1) scrambled eggs with a side of bacon 2) two slices of whole wheat toast, with jam 3) a "superfood" smoothie, whirring up in your blender a peach, an apple, a banana, a kiwi, a cup of strawberries, a cup of blueberries, a few dates, and a handful of goji berries, in unsweetened almond milk 4) a large bowl of oatmeal?

If you chose the plate of scrambled eggs and bacon, I'm worried about you. Clearly you're not reading very closely. You'll probably be consuming about 400 calories without taking in any carbohydrate, the body's primary fuel. About 80-90% of the bacon calories will come from fat, a lot of it saturated. The eggs will be about 66% fat. You'll also get a lot of protein—excessive, unhealthy, potentially carcinogenic animal protein, much of which you will have to piss away (at risk to your bones, from which calcium will be leached to neutralize the acidic protein) because the human body doesn't store protein. And you'll get zero fiber. It's simply not a human meal; it's death on a plate.

The two slices of whole wheat toast with jam will do in a pinch—it's not bad fuel—but it's hardly a very nutritious meal. Its relative healthfulness would depend in part on the ingredients of the bread and of the jam, but let's be generous and assume that it's a bread made entirely from whole grains, and a fruit jam without added sugar. This light meal will provide you with a reasonable tally of about 250 calories—and very few of them from fat, which is good. But, even without added sugar, the jam will be high in natural fruit sugar, and too much of that could lead to a rise in triglycerides and even (especially if much of the sugar comes in the form of fructose) serum cholesterol. (While no plant foods have any appreciable dietary cholesterol, foods that are too fatty or too high in sugar—particularly fructose—can cause your liver to overproduce cholesterol.) Make sure when buying bread to get whole grain flour—you want the ingredient list to say "whole wheat," rather than "wheat"—but even whole grain breads are, like all flour products, calorie-dense. This kind of meal or snack is certainly allowed on the Fuel Plus Fortification plan, but it's less than optimal.

What about that superfood smoothie? Hard to imagine more nutritional goodness in a single glass, right?

Unfortunately, no. If you add up the calories from all the fruit, plus the almond milk, you may have just made yourself a 500-calorie drink. One risk to drinking smoothies stems from the fact that the sugar in the fruit becomes separated from the fiber, leading to a rush of sugar into your bloodstream. Further, by bypassing the process of chewing your food, you have undermined its digestion. And from a weight-loss perspective, the real risk is that there is far less satiety resulting from a pureed drink than from eating whole foods. You would be unlikely to eat an apple, a banana, a kiwi, a cup of strawberries, a cup of blueberries, a few dates, and some goji berries for breakfast. But blend them together and pour them in a glass and you can drink them all very easily, yet still probably not feel full, and then find yourself putting a couple of slices of bread in the toaster to achieve satiety.

Here's what Dr. Caldwell Esselstyn, author of Prevent and Reverse Heart Disease, has to say on the subject: "Avoid smoothies. When the fiber is pureed, it is not chewed and does not have the opportunity to mix with the facultative anaerobic bacteria which reside in the crypts and grooves of our tongue. These bacteria are capable of reducing the nitrates in green leafy vegetables to nitrites in the mouth. When the nitrites are swallowed, they are further reduced by gastric acid to nitric oxide, which may now enter the nitric oxide pool. Furthermore, when chewing fruit, the fructose is bound to fiber and absorption is safe and slow. On the other hand, when fruit is blenderized, the fructose is separated from the fiber and the absorption is very rapid through the stomach. This rapid absorption tends to injure the liver, glycates protein and injures the endothelial cells." [1]

There are some who disagree with Dr. Esselstyn on this score, and claim that the blending of fruits and vegetables makes their nutrients even more bio-available than they would be if chewed. I personally trust Dr. Esselstyn's perspective. I think it's fair to conclude that smoothies can serve as an occasional treat, but certainly if you rely on them as daily fuel, you run the risks that Dr. Esselstyn highlights. It's good to keep in mind as well that green smoothies, made from greens like spinach or kale, or perhaps lightly sweetened with one fruit, will be far less caloric than fruit smoothies. It's also possible, and preferable, to blend less fully and leave the smoothie a little bit chunky. Still, as a general rule, you want to chew your food, not drink it; it's a mistake to make smoothies a staple of your diet.

Your ideal source of breakfast energy is in fact the large bowl of oatmeal. It will have about 150 calories, around 15% of which will come from fat. It will provide about 5 grams of healthy plant protein, and plenty of fiber. You will walk away from the meal satiated, and that is a vital key to weight loss. And if that 150 calorie bowl of oatmeal doesn't fill you up, you can always make a bigger bowl of oatmeal, without concerning yourself with calories at all.

This is your primary key to nutrition and weight-loss: *understanding what our natural human fuel is.* Dr. John McDougall (www.drmcdougall.com) is a visionary pioneer in the plant-based food movement who has established one central priority for his patients and his followers: ensuring that the bulk of their calories should come from a certain class of foods, and the word Dr. McDougall likes to use for those foods is "starch."

Now, as Dr. McDougall well knows, that's a charged word, because most people think of white flour pasta and donuts and bread when they think of "starch," and so they think of starch as something to avoid, especially when concerned about weight loss. What Dr. McDougall boldly calls "starch" is what nutritionists have traditionally called "complex carbohydrate," a phrase seemingly designed to mystify laymen. But Dr. McDougall is right that the word "starch" is the scientifically accurate term for the foods that he recommends form the basis of our diet: potatoes and sweet potatoes, whole grains (rice, wheat, buckwheat, barley, corn, millet, oats, rye, etc.), legumes (beans, peas, lentils), squashes and root vegetables. More importantly, he's right on the merits: these *are* the foods that are natural human fuel. And he's right that by choosing this natural human fuel instead of using animal foods as a source of fuel, your odds are high of escaping the chronic diseases that plague Western societies: heart disease, diabetes, obesity, hypertension, and autoimmune diseases.

To explain why starch is the preeminent fuel for the human body, let me make an analogy to the drought currently plaguing California. Yes, California needs rain, but even more than that, California needs snow. While a heavy summer storm would bring welcome rain to California, the atmospheric temperature would likely be too high for it to bring snow to its Sierra Nevada mountains, and so most of that rain will not be captured. But a winter storm, with underlying cold temperatures, will bring snow that will add to the mountain snowpack, and that mountain snowpack will melt in the spring and replenish the state's reservoirs. Winter storms have a more lasting effect on providing the water that California needs.

When you eat fruit, you're getting a quick charge of energy comparable to a summer storm. When you eat starches, you're adding to your personal snowpack, your energy stores (otherwise known as glycogen). The body will convert that energy to glucose when it needs to.

To extend the analogy, when you blend your fruit, you're getting a flash flood. And when you eat meat and dairy, you're just getting slush.

I tell you as a reluctant expert in dieting, never has adopting a diet been easier than when I embarked on one based on healthy, starchy foods. And never has one been more effective or satisfying. In fact, I never thought of it as a diet at all, just a lifestyle. And I don't think of it as a particularly exotic lifestyle—it's just eating human food. Which, I realize now, I actually hadn't done for the first thirty-six years of my life. There are billions of people around the world—usually the world's less affluent populations—who have made staples like rice and wheat and corn and potatoes the mainstay of their diet, and they do not suffer from the diseases like obesity, heart disease, and type 2 diabetes that plague the affluent West.

As Dr. McDougall summarizes it in "The Starch Solution," "Throughout civilization and around the world, six foods have provided our primary fuel: barley, corn, millet, potatoes, rice, and wheat." [2] He further points out how the fact that human saliva contains more starch-digesting enzyme (amylase) than the saliva of other primates helped allow us, in effect, to conquer the world: "Their limited ability to utilize starch confined chimpanzees and other great apes to tropical jungles around the equator, where they found abundant fruits and perishable vegetables all year long to meet their caloric needs. It was our ability to digest and meet our energy needs with starch that allowed us to migrate north and south and inhabit the entire planet." [3]

Dr. McDougall's emphasis on choosing the correct fuel for the body is surely the most important lesson one can learn on the road to health. But it's hardly the only lesson. Dr. Esselstyn, who has saved the lives of so many patients with heart disease, stresses the importance of fighting inflammatory conditions in the body with foods high in antioxidant capacity (sometimes referred to as the Oxygen Radical Absorbance Capacity, or ORAC value): "Nothing beats the ORAC value of green leafy vegetables....So for patients with heart disease...I've got to get rid of that oxidative cauldron. So, we want them to have a green leafy vegetable the size of your fist after it has been cooked in boiling water five-and-a-half to six minutes so it's nice and tender....How often do I want that? Six times a day. Alongside your breakfast cereal. Again a mid-morning snack. Again with your luncheon sandwich. Again a mid-afternoon snack. Again at dinner time. And god I adore it when you have that evening snack of kale. What you are doing is...you're taking this disease, and you're bathing, you're basking that cauldron of inflammation with nature's most powerful anti-oxidants all day long." [4]

Dr. Esselstyn further emphasizes chewing your greens thoroughly, so that the nitrates present in the greens are reduced by the bacteria in the mouth to nitrites, and later in the stomach will be reduced by gastric acid to nitric oxide, the health-generating compound that keeps our blood vessels dilated (and, by the way, also acts as nature's Viagra).

But wait a minute. Dr. McDougall emphasizes structuring your diet around potatoes, corn, and rice, and now here comes Dr. Esselstyn recommending that we eat kale, spinach, and other greens all day long. How many calories can there possibly be in a small serving of steamed or boiled greens? Twenty? Doesn't that contradict Dr. McDougall's approach?

No, it complements it. Dr. McDougall chooses to emphasize fuel; Dr. Esselstyn chooses to emphasize what I am calling *fortification*, by which I mean the foods we should eat not for their caloric value, not to fill us up, but for their protective properties. These are foods that build up our immune defenses, improve our circulation, lower our cholesterol, clear away toxins, and disrupt tumor formation. And while steamed greens may have pride of place right at the top of that list, it's a long, varied, and wonderful list of foods that includes virtually all fruit, all vegetables, fungi (mushrooms), herbs and spices, seaweed, and fermented plant foods. And the more you look into the wonderful, health-giving, life-sustaining properties of all these foods, the more certain you become that eating an herbivorous diet is nature's plan for humans, as you will not be able to find a single comparative benefit to found anywhere in the entire misbegotten kingdom of animal foods.

To return for a moment to the quiz that began this chapter, there's an even better choice for the ideal dinner, and the ideal breakfast, that I did not present earlier: serve your burrito (fuel) with the colorful raw salad (fortification) and the side of steamed broccoli (more fortification). Have your big bowl of oatmeal (fuel) topped with organic blueberries and cinnamon (fortification).

That's the Fuel Plus Fortification plan. Your *fuel* takes the form of satisfying foods (many considered "comfort foods") like potatoes, sweet potatoes, rice, corn, buckwheat, oats, whole grain bread and pasta, beans, and lentils. Your *fortification* can be found in the whole universe of colorful fruits and vegetables, mushrooms, and herbs and spices that add variety to every meal. Don't neglect either side of the equation. You won't feel satisfied, and your body won't function efficiently, unless you choose the right fuel. And you won't be protecting your health optimally, and you will risk being bored by your food, unless you fortify your meals with nature's glorious, generally low-calorie, endless bounty of nutrient-dense fruits, vegetables, and fungi.

Of course, the foods that serve us best as fuel—such foods as potatoes and sweet potatoes—are rich in nutrients as well. Let's not sell them short. But by combining them with a variety of foods that have a range of nutrients and are minimally caloric, you can achieve optimal nutrition.

As long as we follow Dr. McDougall's advice and choose the right fuel, the opportunity to protect and improve our health with these nutrient-dense foods is staggering. Population studies have demonstrated repeatedly that people who eat five servings or more of fruits and vegetables have about half the risk of developing many types of cancer. [5] And yet only 14% of Americans eat the recommended five servings per day of fruits and vegetables (two fruits and three vegetables). [6] And that's while counting French fries as a vegetable! According to the CDC, the average American actually eats 1.1 fruits per day and 1.6 vegetables per day. [7] The Produce for Better Health Foundation paints an even bleaker picture, reporting less than one fruit consumed per day by Americans and barely more than one vegetable—and this is including canned fruits and vegetables and French fries. [8]

There are many reasons for these appalling statistics, among them the "food deserts" that exist in many of the nation's urban areas, where fresh produce is nearly impossible to obtain. But however you slice it, this is an incredible indictment of the nation often considered the richest in the world. Clearly, we are not rich by the metric of feeding our population. Imagine an African population of chimpanzees, our closest relatives, that could only manage to eat one fruit and a few leaves per day. It would be a doomed population.

We really need to step back for a moment and marvel at what has become of us. We are certainly the most powerful nation on earth. And yet our population has made itself extraordinarily sick and vulnerable by failing to eat the very foods that protect us from disease. Instead, the bulk of our calories are coming from substances that aren't even remotely related to human food. Animal "foods" and processed "foods" are a poor excuse for nutrition, and they are responsible for the chronic diseases plaguing Americans, including of course the one I suffered from for so long, obesity.

By the way, the "recommended" five or more daily servings of fruits and vegetables that the majority of Americans fail to obtain is a pretty pathetic, low-ball recommendation. I eat ten or more such servings per day, and I'm not a big eater.

One meta-study concluded, "Among the dietary factors that are most clearly linked to cancer, a large number of population-based studies have consistently shown that individuals who eat five servings or more of fruits and vegetables daily have approximately half the risk of developing a wide variety of cancer types, particularly those of the gastrointestinal tract." [9] Now either you believe there's something magical about the number five, or you can extrapolate from an understanding of the underlying mechanism at work and conclude that, since fruits and vegetables contain antioxidants that militate against inflammation and cancer causation, the more fruits and vegetables you eat (within reason), the more protection you will get. Therefore, your risk of developing cancer can likely be cut by much more than half, especially if, while eating more than five servings per day of fruits and vegetables, you also totally eliminate animal foods, with their cancer-causing, sulfuric protein. There's no reason to stop at five fruits and vegetables per day; it's easy enough to surpass that number by noon.

How important is the number of servings of fruits and vegetables consumed per day? Well, let's look at Chronic Obstructive Pulmonary Disease (COPD), which comprises emphysema and chronic bronchitis; these are conditions that tend to worsen over time. In the first decade of this century, a study was conducted in Thessaly, Greece, of 120 people who suffer from COPD [10]; half were asked to eat a mere *one extra serving* per day of fruits or vegetables; the control group was not asked to change its diet. Over a period of three years, as might be expected, the control group's health deteriorated. But the lung function of the group eating the additional fruit or vegetable daily actually improved slightly. One can only imagine how much more impressive the results might have been if the intervention group ate, say, five or ten more fruits and vegetables per day.

Researchers prove over and over again the restorative benefits of fruits and vegetables, and yet this approach to healing is rarely mentioned by American doctors who every day treat a flood of patients with chronic diseases such as heart disease, type 2 diabetes, or hypertension— all usually caused by diet, not by genes.

Here's an amazing study to demonstrate the significant role of fortification in a healthy diet. Esophageal cancer is a tough cancer to be diagnosed with; according to the American Cancer Society, the percentage of five year survival after being diagnosed with esophageal cancer is 38% for localized cancer to the esophagus (and much less if the cancer has already spread beyond the esophagus). [11] Wouldn't it be wonderful if there were a food that could prevent the development of esophageal cancer? Well, a clinical study demonstrates that there is such a food. Is it fried chicken? No. Pork bellies? Wrong again. Maybe a nice sharp cheddar cheese? No. It is in fact—surprise!—a plant food. Strawberries.

Thirty-six patients with dysplastic premalignant esophageal lesions received freeze-dried strawberry powder for six months. At the end of six months, the treatment reversed the lesions of twenty-nine of those thirty-six patients. [12]

Imagine if a drug company could come up with a compound that worked even half that well on esophageal cancer. Its stock would sky-rocket. But the compound in this case was strawberries, which cannot be owned by a drug company, so that may be why you haven't heard about this study.

Tumors cannot grow without a blood supply. It turns out that certain compounds interrupt the angiogenesis of blood vessels that support tumors. Where do you suppose those compounds are found? Chicken nuggets? Whole milk yogurt? Goat cheese? Egg salad? No, it turns out, shockingly, that these compounds are known as *phytochemicals*—*phyto* being Greek for "plant"—and the capacity to disrupt tumor blood supply has been found in specific phytochemicals present in tea, spices, fruit, and beans. [13]

Tumors also thrive on an excess of one particular amino acid: methionine. You may have heard of dogs that can actually sniff out tumors; they are able to do so because tumors transform methionine into gaseous compounds. What kind of diet is low in methionine? A vegan diet. Methionine is a sulfuric amino acid abundant in the proteins in flesh foods.

Breast cancer cell proliferation has been shown in *in vitro* studies to be halted by the action of single food that inhibits the enzymes that tumors use to make estrogen to fuel their growth. What is that food? If you guessed pastrami, you're off my Christmas list. It is, in fact, mush-rooms. As few as five button mushrooms per day may do the trick to protect women from breast cancer. [14]

The author Dan Buettner has studied and written books about what he calls "Blue Zones"—regions of the world with the greatest longevity, where people live to 100 or more at many times the rate that they do in the United States. He found many characteristics that these people share in common, some of them cultural, but on the nutritional front he found one food that they all seemed to eat in far greater amounts than we do in the United States. What do you think that food was?

Something exotic perhaps? Octopus? Ostrich? *Escargot*? No, in fact, it was the lowly bean. Buettner recommends eating a cup of beans per day. [15]

Bile acids are synthesized in the liver and serve a number of functions, but excess bile acids can be a factor in Crohn's disease, colorectal cancer, and heart disease. Optimally they are bound by compounds in certain foods before they can do you any harm. What kind of foods do you think have been demonstrated to play that bile-binding role most efficiently? If you guessed hot dogs, you may need to be institutionalized. In fact, the foods that excel in this regard are collard greens, kale, mustard greens, broccoli, and cabbage—and to get their full bile-acid-binding effect, steam them. [16]

Nitrates occur naturally in some kinds of food, which our enzymes or bacteria in the mouth turn into nitrites (two oxygen atoms bonded to a nitrogen atom, instead of three), and then, as Dr. Esselstyn has pointed out, they get converted into nitric oxide, which is so crucial to arterial health and to maintaining a healthy blood pressure. Which kinds of foods are naturally high in nitrate? If you guessed *steak tartare*, I'm sorry, you're clearly an idiot. The champions are Swiss chard, basil, beet greens, spring greens, butter lettuce, arugula, cilantro, and rhubarb. [17]

Meats are, however, often preserved with nitrites, which gives a red color to cured meat. So is that just as good? Hardly. When cooked at high heat (as meat must be, as it is always rife with pathogens), those nitrites are converted not into healthy nitric oxide but rather into carcinogenic nitrosamines.

The examples are endless of the role that plant foods (including mushrooms, technically fungi) can play in fortifying our bodies against disease and decline. Literally thousands of nutritional studies have demonstrated reason to believe in the health-promoting effects of fruits, vegetables, whole grains, legumes, herbs, and spices.

While it's hard to prove a negative, let me go out on a limb and state what I believe to be true: *I don't believe there's a single legitimate nutritional study ever conducted that has demonstrated a single health-promoting effect of any single animal food.* Now, to be clear, there are studies that make the case for fish, for example—but only by comparing those who eat a certain number of servings of fish to those on the standard American diet, never by comparing fish-eaters to those practicing a healthful, low-fat, vegan diet. There are studies that compare one lousy diet to another and conclude that dairy or eggs or some other deadly food appears to have some benefits. But you'd think that, if there were really any legitimate case to be made for any animal food—let's say Swiss cheese—there would be a very easy way to prove it. Set up a control group on a low-fat, whole-foods, starch-based vegan diet, and compare it to another group that eats a similar diet plus X number of servings per day of Swiss cheese, and find the health metric that improves with the Swiss cheese.

That study has never been done, and it never will be done. There are no studies that have ever been designed or ever will be designed to show the benefit of any animal food by comparing those who consume that food with a control group on a low-fat, whole-foods, starch-based vegan diet.

No animal food producer is going to pay for that study. And, most likely, no scientist would believe so strongly in the benefit of any animal food that he or she would design such a study to try to legitimately prove the benefit.

And yet studies have been done, as we have seen, of people on pretty lousy diets, and they just add one fruit or vegetable and, remarkably enough, show improvement.

Our goal here, of course, isn't to just add one fruit or vegetable to a lousy diet; it's to think about fuel plus fortification at every meal and thereby eat an optimal diet. Here are some meal ideas to help you accomplish that goal.

For breakfast:
Oatmeal with organic strawberries, blueberries, raspberries, blackberries, grapes, or goji berries. Or any other fruit: apple, pear, banana, kiwi, etc. (Note: sweeten your oatmeal with fruit, not with sugar. Sugar is an addictive substance that adds empty calories and does more harm than good to the body. In all its forms but whole foods—like fruit—minimize the sugar in your diet.) Health tip: add some oat bran to your oat flakes for added fiber, and watch your cholesterol numbers go down.

Raw steel-cut oats with persimmons.

A bowl of buckwheat, plus a fruit or two.

Corn grits, plus a fruit or two.

A hot wheat-based cereal (Wheatena or couscous), with added fruit.

A whole grain cold cereal, low in sugar (try to find one sweetened just with fruit juice), with an unsweetened plant milk (almond, soy, hemp, rice), topped with berries.

Rice or buckwheat with steamed greens. (There is no law against steamed greens in the morning.)

For lunch:
A bean-and-rice burrito (made on a corn or wheat tortilla), with added tomatoes. On the side, a salad and/or steamed greens.

A bean salad.

Miso soup with rice and mushrooms.

Lentil soup with potatoes and carrots.

A tempeh (fermented soy) sandwich on whole grain bread, with lettuce and tomato and whatever condiments you wish. Steamed greens and/or a salad on the side.

Same as above but make it a portobello "burger" on whole grain bread. Or any "burger" made from beans, lentils, or whole grains (added nuts and seeds acceptable).

Wild rice with steamed vegetables. Or sautee your vegetables in water or tamari.

Penne pasta in a marinara sauce with mushrooms, and steamed broccoli and spinach, topped with a nut-based "parmesan."

Hummus (try to find an oil-free version, or make an oil-free version yourself) on rice crackers or whole grain bread or cucumber slices. Salad on the side.

For dinner:

Red lentil chili (see recipe section), with steamed greens.

Quinoa Curry Bowl (see recipe section)

Pasta with basil pesto, with steamed asparagus.

Vegetable casserole (see recipe section)

Mung bean curry (see recipe section)

Pinto bean enchiladas with mushrooms

Baked tofu and sweet potato with salad

Potato leek soup, corn chowder, or black bean soup

These are the kinds of meals that will leave you satisfied, and that, by combining starches with nutrient-dense, low-calorie vegetables, will fortify your body against disease.

Now where do I get off, you may rightly ask, creating a diet? After all, I'm not a doctor, nutritionist, or research scientist. I'm just a regular guy who was morbidly obese and lost half his weight. Am I qualified to suggest that everyone follow my own dietary regimen?

Well, it isn't my own; I make no claims to breakthrough originality. There's scarcely a dime's worth of difference between what I'm calling Fuel Plus Fortification, and the McDougall Plan, or for that matter the dietary regime recommended by Dr. Esselstyn and any number of other leaders of the plant-based food movement. If I have something to contribute, it's merely a new *framework* for viewing and incorporating the ideas of these great pioneers of plant-based eating.

I found that, for myself, designing meals that combine healthy starch with a wide range of nutrient-dense, low-calorie vegetables, and snacking on fruits, or creating fruit-based desserts (without added sugar), helped me lose half my weight consistently and easily without ever getting bored.

If that framework can help others, I gladly offer it up.

CHAPTER 4

The Movie That Changed My Life

t was Memorial Day weekend, 2013. I was 258 pounds—not quite the heaviest I'd ever been, but within shooting distance. I was already making up my mind to embark again on another of my endless carb-restricting diets, basing my diet around chicken, fish, and vegetables. I would totally abstain from "carbs"—pasta, bread, rice, and sugar. This time, I promised myself, I wouldn't quit after losing twenty or thirty pounds; I would stick with it. Of course, I'd made that promise to myself before.

I was feeling the usual cognitive dissonance I felt whenever diving back into one of these high-protein diets. It stemmed from the fact that these diets never quite made sense to me. I'm a rational guy; science and math were my best subjects in school. If I don't understand the logic behind what I'm doing, that gnaws at me a little bit. Now I had read books promoting these meat-centered diets, and knew from experience that losing twenty or thirty pounds on them was easily achievable, but still, I never quite grasped the logic behind the thesis that eating fatty flesh foods like chicken and fish (much less the hamburger and steak that I was also allowed on these plans) should be the key to losing weight. Even "lean" meats, I knew, were still far fattier than the "carbs" I needed to avoid. I could never quite figure out why that trade-off should work, but I assumed that there must be something about diet that defied logic, or at any rate that outstripped my scientific understanding; after all, everyone knew that avoiding "carbs" was the only reliable way to lose weight. And it had worked for me before, sort of.

Claire and I sat down to watch a documentary. I'm something of a documentary buff—I was a film major in college—and Claire often enjoys them as well. In any case, she humors me. I didn't know anything about the choice that happened to cross my eye, a film called *Forks Over Knives*. I simply stumbled upon it that evening as I browsed the options under the category *Documentary* on Amazon Prime Video. I think I noticed in my search that the subject was nutrition and health but beyond that I had no clue what it was about. I hadn't read any reviews or spoken to anyone who had seen it. I figured there was no harm in streaming it; if we didn't like it after fifteen minutes, we could move on to something else. I sure as hell wasn't looking to change my life; I was just looking to be entertained for 90 minutes and maybe learn a thing or two.

If you haven't already seen the film, I encourage you to do so, and also to visit the website (http://www.forksoverknives.com), where the *Forks Over Knives* (FOK) diet is described (and, again, I see no real difference between the FOK diet and The McDougall Plan or Fuel Plus Fortification or a diet centered around the Four Food Groups promoted by the Physicians Committee for Responsible Medicine). Here's how the film is synopsized on the *Forks Over Knives* website: "*Forks Over Knives* examines the profound claim that most, if not all, of the degenerative diseases that afflict us can be controlled, or even reversed, by rejecting our present menu of animal-based and processed foods. The major storyline in the film traces the personal journeys of a pair of pioneering yet under-appreciated researchers, Dr. T. Colin Campbell and Dr. Caldwell Esselstyn." [1]

Watching that film was truly a ninety-minute-long *Eureka!* moment. Here was what seemed to me a revolutionary idea: instead of eating fatty animal products, eat less caloric, less fatty foods from the plant kingdom, fill yourself up on starchy foods (that I love), like potatoes, and stop worrying about protein! I had never heard before that animal protein could be carcinogenic, and that ingesting too much protein could be harmful. Man, that was a revelation. It made me a little indignant that I had never come across this information before.

As I watched the evidence mount that animal foods were the leading cause of obesity and diabetes, something clicked in me. I realized that indeed it made no sense that fatty meat, butter, and oil should be the keys to losing weight. Not only was it illogical; it was untrue. I realized that putting oneself into an unhealthy state of ketosis by depriving oneself of carbohydrate was patently nutty. The comparisons of health metrics between cultures that ate a starch-based diet versus the animal-based Western diet sealed the case. I realized that I had been duped for so many years, and I was astonished that I hadn't been exposed to the sensible ideas expressed in the film before. I was thirty-six years old, and this was the first time I was hearing about the correct, natural way humans should eat.

Not only did the premise make sense that eating a low-fat, plant-based diet led to weight loss, but the film made the greater claim that it was the key to avoiding heart disease, diabetes, and so many of the other diseases plaguing our society.

Claire and I knew only a few vegetarians, and they didn't seem particularly healthy; they were not particularly good advertisements for the vegetarian diet. We didn't know any vegans. I suppose that was one reason that I had never considered going on a vegetarian or vegan diet. Another reason was actually linguistic: both words start with "veg," and when I thought of those diets, I thought of eating vegetables all day long—and I was never a big fan of a lot of vegetables. So, I couldn't imagine myself eating romaine lettuce and asparagus all day. It seemed like it would be a very hungry existence. But after watching the film, which demonstrated the health improvements and weight-loss of several individuals who switched to plant-based eating, I realized that a diet could be constructed around foods like whole grains, beans, peas, lentils, potatoes, corn, and fruit—not just vegetables and salad greens.

Claire and I both knew that a lot of people we knew would consider the idea of going on a vegan diet extreme. Then again, I was well aware that weighing 258 pounds was also pretty extreme. So we both agreed to try a vegan diet for thirty days and see what happens. It was the opposite, after all, of everything I had tried before, and since everything I had tried before had ultimately failed, maybe trying the opposite approach made sense.

We announced our intention to our family and closest friends, so they would be aware not to cook any animal foods for us and would understand any unusual, new food-related behaviors on our part. Generally, everyone was curious but supportive. And I'm pretty sure everyone expected that this gambit would be short-lived (after all, everything I had tried before had been short-lived, and all progress reversed). In the meantime, we learned to field and humor the usual misguided questions about where we would get our protein and calcium.

In the first month, I lost about 14 pounds. It turned out that a vegan diet wasn't at all hard to follow. I found lots of vegan burgers and ready-made or processed vegan foods at the local Whole Foods. There were even plenty of vegan options at restaurants, especially if they were reasonably upscale restaurants seeking to please their customers. Usually the chef would work with you even if there wasn't an option on the menu. Contacting restaurants in advance of showing up always proved a good idea. And if a group of friends was going to a restaurant that wasn't particularly vegan-friendly, we would still join them, and try to create a meal from side dishes or eat a snack first so we wouldn't get hungry. We weren't about to let our new diet separate us from our friends; going out, after all, is about more than the food. From the start, we wanted to demonstrate that we can go anywhere anyone goes, that ours is a perfectly mainstream way to live, and that we don't want to be a pain-in-the-ass.

I immediately began reading all kinds of wonderful books that helped me understand the science behind my new diet: *The Starch Solution* by Dr. John McDougall; *The China Study* and *Whole* by T. Colin Campbell and Thomas Campbell; *Prevent and Reverse Heart Disease* by Dr. Caldwell Esselstyn; *The Engine 2 Diet* and *My Beef with Meat* by Rip Esselstyn (son of Dr. Esselstyn); *The Pleasure Trap* by Doug Lisle; *Diet for a New America* by John Robbins; *Keep it Simple, Keep it Whole* by Dr. Alona Pulde and Dr. Matthew Lederman; *21-Day Weight-Loss Kickstart* by Dr. Neal Barnard, *Food Choice and Sustainability* by Dr. Richard Oppenlander; and *Unprocessed* by Chef AJ.

Month after month, about twelve to fifteen pounds would come off, and at first it felt like I hardly needed to make much of an effort. I was succeeding just by keeping anything animal-derived off my plate. I was still eating foods prepared with oils, and a lot of processed vegan food, such as a vegan version of macaroni and cheese (with the cheese made from processed soy and oils).

My initial goal was to get down to my wedding weight of 204. I surpassed that goal after five months.

After six months, and below 200 pounds, I decided to step up my game. By that point, I had read enough to know that processed foods, even if vegan, were not particularly healthy, and that oil was not a health food. Oil is 100% fat, and so it's illogical to expect it to make a positive contribution to weight-loss. Cutting out oils was, for me, the most challenging part of the diet, as so many packaged foods you buy in the supermarket are prepared with oil. And it's of course very difficult to get meals in restaurants that are prepared oil-free. So, cutting out oils meant preparing more of our meals at home using whole foods, rather than relying on processed foods and restaurant fare. Doing so re-accelerated my weight loss.

The next major goal that I achieved was to reach the milestone weight of 158 by Memorial Day, 2014. That meant that I had lost 100 pounds in a year's time.

Gradually, I began to emphasize getting in my share of fortification foods every day—usually in the form of fruits and steamed vegetables. I found, too, that by steaming my greens and other vegetables lightly, that meant I would be chewing more, and it seemed that the more I chewed my food, the less I felt that I needed to eat. I began to eat about two to three servings of fruit per day, and six to eight servings of vegetables. I succeeded almost completely in avoiding added oils, sugar, and salt.

As my diet improved, unhealthy foods that used to taste good to me lost their appeal. French fries tasted terribly greasy. A sip of soft drink tasted way too sugary. Restaurant food often tasted too salty.

If I was having a meal with a calorie-dense food like pasta alongside low-calorie fortification foods like steamed spinach and a salad, I would make sure that I ate all of the fortification foods first, so that if I became full before cleaning my plate and needed to leave any part of the meal over, it would be the more calorie-dense food.

I ate whenever I was hungry, but I tried not to let myself eat when I was not. And I began a regimen of daily swimming.

My weight-loss continued, month after month. Obviously, it's harder to lose weight after you've already lost 100 pounds and you're closer to your natural, healthy weight, but still the pounds came off, four or five per month until I hit my low at 125 in November, 2014. I currently fluctuate in the range of 130-135, and have done so consistently for the last year or so.

Claire and I would cook our "fuel" food in large batches, making great quantities of, say, red lentil chili, chick pea curry (we like spicy food), any kind of rice dish, split pea soup, or potatoes, so that we didn't have to cook that often and this whole new way of eating became more convenient. There was always something to grab in the fridge if we got hungry. And so we learned how to make our new dietary plan extremely convenient and easy.

My go-to desserts or snacks became watermelon, cherries, grapes, peaches, pineapple, or plums. And sometimes a handful of nuts.

Finally, here was a diet that wasn't an ordeal; instead, it was a pleasure, and I was discovering new foods all the time along the way.

After losing half my weight, my story was told in such media outlets as *CNN* and *The Globe*, as well as on Dr. McDougall's website. [2] I began attending conferences in the plant-based food movement and met many of its leading lights. And now I myself create and organize conferences as part of our nonprofit, Remedy Food Project (www.remedyfood.org).

I have begun to meet countless people who have had their health and their lives dramatically improved, as mine was, by renouncing animal products. I'm just another face in that happy crowd.

There's another side to the success of this way of eating: psychologically, it came as a great relief to me. I've always been a great animal-lover. Dogs and cats, for sure, but all animals as well. And, in all the years that I was eating meat, I was troubled by the implicit violence it involved, a form of violence that was hidden from me as a consumer but that didn't require too much insight to recognize was part of the bargain. I would buy the meat, and I would be entirely removed from the acts of confinement and slaughter that produced it; the final product would be disguised as much as possible so as not to remind me of the living, breathing animal that was its source.

All states have animal protection laws that protect dogs and cats from cruel owners who would subject them to physical pain. All of us would all condemn in the strongest terms someone who intentionally inflicted harm on a dog. Dogs, after all, have central nervous systems and feel pain. But, of course, so do pigs and cows—and yet farm animals are exempt from animal protection laws. A pig can be kept its whole life in a crate so small that it can't turn around. Cows likewise are housed on cement and treated in ways that would be considered horribly abusive and would lead to immediate arrests of their owners if they were dogs and not "food animals." Not to mention, of course, that they are cruelly slaughtered in the end, their throats slit and their bodies suspended upside down as they bleed to death, often while still kicking.

But we turn a blind eye to the horrors others inflict on these animals on our behalf because they are "food." I had always accepted that discomfiting reality because I saw no alternative to it. Yes, it was a shame that cows and pigs and chickens had to suffer so that I could live, but after all, they were "food," and, as much as I love animals, I've always valued human life above all, and so if these animals had to suffer miserable lives and die miserable deaths so that I and my fellow humans could eat and live, there was nothing that could be done about it. Such was the inherent conflict involved in being a lover of animals who so often had dead ones on his plate. I tried not to think about it.

So, it was liberating to realize that animals are not in fact human food after all. That led to the terrible conclusion that all the suffering we inflict on them is entirely unnecessary, and the wonderful conclusion that we can finally stop it if only we muster the will.

Since animal agriculture is also the largest single contributor to human induced (or "anthropogenic") greenhouse gases and climate change, and the single greatest threat to our environment and to sustaining human life (and that of other species) on this planet, it is imperative that we muster that will. Although the United Nation's Food and Agriculture Organization (FAO) shocked the world with its 2006 report, "Livestock's Long Shadow," in which it calculated livestock's contribution to global greenhouse gases at 18%, more than all forms of transportation combined, that report has since been questioned by some as being too conservative. In their article, "Livestock and Climate Change," researchers Robert Goodland and Jeff Anhang reported that "...livestock and their byproducts actually account for *at least* (emphasis theirs) ...51%of annual worldwide GHG (greenhouse gas) emissions."

According to the International Livestock Research Institute, livestock now use more than 45% of the entire ice free terrestrial land on Earth, or nearly 80% of all land used for agriculture on Earth. Regenerating forest on much of this land is the best and really the only hope for reversing climate change; to do so would be far more significant than increasing the fuel mileage of our vehicles.

Of course, much of that forest has been cleared precisely to raise livestock. 26% of land worldwide is dedicated to grazing livestock, and one-third of arable land is used to grow feed. [3]

And so the suffering we inflict on livestock is far worse than unnecessary; it is wildly destructive, not only to our own health but to the health of the planet.

In addition to our own health, the welfare of animals we treat as commodities and the impact on our planet, there is also the not insignificant effect that the standard Western diet has on our economy. Obesity, to name just one problem, contributes to a range of diseases from diabetes to cancer, and the costs of those diseases have a pernicious effect on federal and state budgets as well as productivity in the private economy, and of course health insurance rates. We all pay for those who choose to eat the rich Western diet and thereby become fat and sick. In the south, where I live, *self-reported* rates of obesity (and let's be honest, if we're depending on those who readily admit they are obese, these rates are low) for 2013 were 30-35% in Georgia, South Carolina, Alabama and Tennessee, 25-30% in North Carolina and Florida, and more than 35% in the state of Mississippi. (CDC)

As of 2012, the CDC reports that half of all adults have one or more chronic condition. One in four has two or more chronic conditions. In 2010, 7 of the top 10 causes of death in this country were chronic, preventable diseases. Here's the real kicker: 84% of all health care spending in 2006 was spent on the 50% of our population who have one or more chronic conditions that can be prevented or controlled with diet. The total cost of heart disease and stroke in 2010 was 315 billion dollars. On diabetes? 245 billion. And medical costs linked to obesity were 128 billion dollars in 2003. [4] (CDC) (All of the above, reference http://www.cdc.gov/chronicdisease/overview/)

Most of us value such entitlements as Medicare. But are we entitled to make dietary choices that overburden the system so that it won't be around in the future for our children?

Just think how much money could be saved if Americans knew just how powerful diet can be in one's health. The sick would save money; their insurance companies would save money; we would ALL save money. If our healthcare system was truly used as it was intended – for broken bones and bleeding – and was not clogged with lifestyle-caused chronic diseases, think how much easier it would be for those who are truly in need of urgent care to see a physician. We can keep victims of preventable illnesses out of our hospitals – just by educating them about the power that they hold at the end of their forks.

Let me leave you with one more sobering aspect to consider: your loved ones. You've probably heard the commercials on radio or television selling life insurance – "make sure your loved ones will be taken care of if the unthinkable were to happen." Well, let's take an uncomfortable moment to actually think about "the unthinkable" – death. Unfortunately, we all do have a 100% chance of dying at some point in our lives, but, barring accidental death, when that happens (i.e., from 'natural causes') – is largely up to us.

We all see friends and family members die much too early – how many of those deaths could have been prevented if we were to take obesity, high blood pressure, heart attacks or strokes out of the equation? Before you eat that next artery-clogging cheeseburger, or put that next huge slab of meat on the grill, ask yourself how your spouse, significant other, parent, child, friend or other loved one would feel if you were to simply drop dead? Ask yourself if you're doing all you can to maintain your health and longevity not only for yourself, but for those who would be crushed if you were to perish tomorrow. Is eating 'what tastes good' or is quick and convenient worth shaving a year off your life? What about ten years? Twenty? Is that box of "chicken" nuggets or churned, sweetened, frozen bovine growth excretion (that's ice cream, by the way) really worth all that?

I bring you this message as a man who was once twice the size nature intended him to be. Now I eat a very satisfying diet, with a wide variety of foods, and I am a slender, healthy guy. It's hard to express in words how miraculous this transformation has been for me. I am a new man. I can feel good about the fact that I have dramatically reduced the chances that I will become a burden on my wife and loved ones as I age. And, to be sure, my friends and loved ones are thrilled for me. And, since they know me for who I am—an easygoing guy who doesn't like to preach, who has a live-and-let-live approach to life—I'm sure that most of my friends and loved ones think, "Hey, it's great that Benji has found a diet that works for him, but he must understand that diet is an individual thing and that his diet isn't right for everybody."

Actually, as much as I hate to disappoint my friends and loved ones, I don't believe that for a minute. I believe that, in the main, the diet I practice is absolutely right for everybody. Of course, we all have our individual tastes and preferences about food. But we are all born herbivores, and I believe it is unnatural and antithetical to human health and to planetary health for humans to twist themselves into omnivores, as if we had evolved as members of the bear family instead of as primates.

I believe in science, and there's really no way you can believe in science and evolution and make the case that humans are natural predators and omnivores.

I believe it is a perverse mistake—a mistake that I regret that I made for so long—to eat the flesh of animals and products made from the lactation of other animals.

It is a mistake that I know can be corrected without any great effort. And once corrected, it invariably leads to improved health.

I like to think of myself as living proof of that fact.

RECIPES

MEXICAN STUFFED POTATO
Recipe credit: Chef AJ
(Serves 2)

Ingredients
2 potatoes (any kind – I prefer Yukon Gold)
1 15-oz. can salt-free pinto beans (or 1.5 cups of your favorite beans)
8 oz. frozen corn
Salt-free salsa or pico de gallo to taste
Jalapenos (optional)
Cilantro (optional)

Preparation
Cook potato however you normally would (bake, steam, pressure cook, microwave).
Heat up the corn and beans, stuff the potato with them and top with salsa. Add jalapenos and cilantro, if desired.

SWEET POTATO AND YELLOW SPLIT PEA SOUP
Recipe credit: Chef AJ

(Serves 4-6)

Ingredients
1 lb. yellow split peas
1 large onion, chopped
1 lb. carrots, sliced
1 celery heart, sliced
2 large sweet potatoes, cubed
8 cups boiling water
6-8 cloves garlic, pressed
4 tsp dried parsley
1-2 T salt-free seasoning*
1 tsp dried basil
1 tsp dried oregano
1 tsp celery seed
1 tsp smoked paprika
1 bay leaf
*Chef AJ recommends *Benson's Table Tasty*

Preparation
Place all ingredients in an Electric Pressure Cooker (we prefer the *Instant Pot*). Cook on high for 8 minutes. Alternatively, place all ingredients in a slow cooker and cook on low for 6-8 hours.
Chef's Note: Serve over brown rice and/or raw or cooked spinach and other greens. Or stir in some greens right after releasing the pressure.

CHIPOTLE BEAN BURGERS
Recipe credit: Chef AJ, inspired by a recipe from the Whole Foods Market website
(Serves 24 burgers)

Ingredients
4 cans salt-free black beans rinsed and drained (or 6 cups cooked beans)
4 cups cooked brown rice
4 cups cooked and mashed sweet potato
1 14.5-oz. can, salt-free, fire-roasted tomatoes
1 cup red onion, chopped
8 cloves garlic, minced
1 red bell pepper finely chopped (approx. 1 cup)
1 large carrot finely chopped (approx. 1 cup)
1 bunch cilantro
12 T nutritional yeast
4 T No-salt-added chili powder
1 T smoked paprika
1 T ground cumin
1 tsp chipotle powder

Preparation
Preheat the oven to 400° F. Drain the can of tomatoes and sauté the onion in the liquid until soft. Add the chopped carrot, bell pepper and garlic and sauté until soft and cooked, about 10-15 minutes.
Line a baking sheet with a *Silpat* (a non-stick baking mat) or piece of parchment paper. Combine all ingredients in a large bowl and stir to mix. Chill several hours or overnight. Make patties out of ½ cup of the mixture. Place patties on the baking sheet and bake, for 40-45 minutes.

Flip and bake for another 20-30 minutes. Makes 24 burgers that freeze well.

<u>Chef's Note</u>: Serve with all the fixings, such as sliced tomatoes and onions and salt-free condiments and use large butter lettuce leaves or potato waffles (a small potato, cooked until brown in a waffle iron) as buns.

RED LENTIL CHILI
Recipe credit: Chef AJ

(Serves 4-6)

Ingredients

1 lb. red lentils

8 cups water

2 14.5-oz. cans of salt-free tomatoes, fire-roasted preferred

1 6-oz. can of salt-free tomato paste

1 large onion, chopped

2 large red bell peppers

3 oz. dates (approx. 12 Deglet Noor)

8 cloves of garlic

4 T apple cider vinegar

1½ T parsley flakes

1½ T oregano

1½ T salt-free chili powder

2 tsp smoked paprika

½ tsp chipotle powder (or more to taste)

¼ tsp crushed red pepper flakes (or more to taste)

Chef AJ's Faux Parmesan (recipe follows)

Preparation

Blend the dates, tomatoes, red bell peppers, and garlic in a blender until smooth. Place all remaining ingredients in an *Instant Pot* electric pressure cooker and cook on high for 10 minutes. Alternately, place all ingredients in a slow cooker and cook on low for 6-8 hours.

Chef AJ's Faux Parmesan Ingredients

1 cup slivered or sliced almonds, cashews, or oats

½ cup nutritional yeast

2-3 T Salt-free seasoning (Chef AJ prefers Benson's Table Tasty)

<u>Preparation</u>
Add ingredients to food processor, process to a medium or fine consistency.

<u>Chef's Note:</u> This is delicious served over a baked Yukon Gold potato or brown rice. Recipe may be halved.

LENTIL TOSTADAS WITH CHILI-LIME SLAW
Recipe credit: Chef AJ
(Serves 4-6)

To make the lentil "Taco Meat:"
<u>Ingredients</u>
1 lb. dried lentils (green or black, not red)
4 cups water
2 cups sliced mushrooms
2 cups chopped onion
4 tsp roasted cumin
1 T oregano
2 T chili powder
2 T salt-free seasoning such as *Benson's Table Tasty*
6 cloves garlic, pressed

<u>Preparation</u>
Place all ingredients in the *Instant Pot* electric pressure cooker on high and cook for 8 minutes. Alternatively, place all ingredients in a slow cooker and cook on low for 6-8 hours.

To make the Chili Lime Slaw:
<u>Ingredients</u>
Shredded cabbage (1 medium cabbage head)
½ cup water
½ cup lime juice
½ tsp crushed red pepper flakes (or to taste)

Preparation

Mix together water, lime juice and red pepper flakes. Pour over shredded cabbage and let marinate at least 15 minutes before serving. Drain excess liquid before topping the tostadas.

Assembly

Take one tortilla and lightly swipe with healthy store-bought guacamole or salsa. Heap on the lentil "meat" and top with the chili lime slaw. Garnish with chopped cilantro or chopped scallions, if desired.

HAIL TO THE KALE SALAD REVISITED
Recipe adapted from *Unprocessed* by Chef AJ
(Serves 2-4)

Ingredients
Salad:
2 large heads of curly kale
Chopped almonds
Dressing:
½ cup raw almond butter (unsweetened and unsalted)
1 15-oz. can of cannellini beans (rinsed and drained)
1 cup water
¼ cup fresh lime juice and zest
2 cloves garlic
Fresh peeled ginger (about 1 in. piece)
2 T low-sodium Tamari soy sauce
4 pitted Medjool or 8 Deglet Noor dates (soaked in water if not soft)
½ teaspoon red pepper flakes.

Preparation
In a high-powered blender, combine all dressing ingredients and blend until smooth and creamy. Remove the thick, larger stems from the kale. Chop the kale as finely as you would like it. Pour desired amount of dressing over kale and massage it in with your hands (wearing food service gloves, if desired) until kale begins to soften.

Chef's note: This salad is also delicious with peanut butter instead of the almond butter and when shredded raw beets and carrots are added to it. If you have a dehydrator, dip kale leaves in the dressing and dehydrate for delicious kale chips! If you are allergic to nuts, use tahini (sesame seed paste) or sunflower seed butter in place of nut butter.

GREEN SPLIT PEA SOUP
Recipe credit: Chef AJ

(Serves 4-6)

Ingredients

1 lb. green split peas

1 large onion, chopped

1 lb. carrots, sliced

1 celery heart, sliced

2 large potatoes, cubed

8 cups boiling water

6-8 cloves garlic, pressed

T tsp dried parsley

1-2 T salt-free seasoning such as *Benson's Table Tasty*

1 tsp dried basil

1 tsp dried rosemary

1 tsp dried oregano

1 tsp celery seed

1 tsp smoked paprika

1 bay leaf

Chef AJ's Faux Parmesan to taste (recipe on page XX)

Preparation

Place all ingredients in an *Instant Pot* electric pressure cooker. Cook on high for 8 minutes. Alternatively, place all ingredients in a slow cooker and cook on low for 6-8 hours.

Chef's Note: Serve over brown rice and/or raw or cooked spinach or other greens. Or, stir in some greens right after releasing the pressure.

ENCHILADA STRATA
Recipe credit: Chef AJ
(Serves 4-6)

To make the sauce:
<u>Ingredients</u>
1 red onion, chopped
2 cloves garlic, crushed
1 28-oz. can salt-free tomatoes, fire-roasted preferred
2 T chili powder
1 tsp roasted cumin
3 T arrowroot powder
1½ cups water

<u>Preparation</u>
Place the onion, garlic and liquid in a pot and cook 8-10 minutes until soft. Stir in tomato and spices and cook on low heat for 15 minutes. Add the arrowroot powder to a small amount of cold water and dissolve, then add to sauce and stir until thickened.

To make the filling:
<u>Ingredients</u>
4 cups salt-free salsa [Note: is that easy to find?]
2½ lbs. sweet potatoes, mashed
1 lb. bag frozen roasted corn, defrosted
1 4-oz. can mild green chilies
2 15-oz. cans salt-free black beans, rinsed and drained (or 6 cups of cooked beans)
2 16-oz. bags frozen kale, defrosted with all the liquid squeezed out
12 corn tortillas
Optional garnishes: sliced olives, scallions

Preparation

Peel sweet potatoes and boil or steam until soft. Process in a food processor fitted with the "S" blade until smooth and creamy. Place into a large bowl and stir in the salsa, corn, beans, and kale. Mix well. Using food service gloves is recommended so that everything gets fully incorporated.

Assembly

Preheat oven to 350° F. Cover the bottom of a large baking dish with half of the enchilada sauce. A lasagna pan is recommended. Place 6 tortillas on top of the enchilada sauce and then gently and evenly place the sweet potato mixture on top of the tortillas. Top with the remaining 6 tortillas. Pour the remaining sauce over the tortillas and sprinkle sliced olives, if desired, over the top. Bake for 30 minutes. Sprinkle with scallions if desired.

QUINOA SALAD WITH CURRANTS
Recipe credit: Chef AJ
(Serves 4-6)

Ingredients
2 cups pre-rinsed quinoa (try red or tricolor quinoa for a colorful change of pace)

3 cups water (start with boiling water so it will cook faster)

1 cup lime juice, add zest if using fresh

2 oz. fresh mint, finely chopped

2 oz. parsley, finely chopped

2 oz. scallion, finely chopped

2 cups currants

2 cups pomegranate seeds

8 oz. pistachios, crushed (optional)

Preparation
Place quinoa in the pressure cooker. Cook on high pressure for 2 minutes. Let it come down to pressure for at least 10 minutes. Release any remaining pressure and place the quinoa in a large bowl. Add lime juice, fresh mint, parsley, currants and pomegranate seeds. Mix well. Optional: add pistachio nuts, crushed.

Chef's Note: For finely chopped herbs, chop them in the food processor fitted with the "S" blade. Make sure that both the food processor and the herbs are completely dry. If there is any water or moisture, you will get pesto!

When pomegranate seeds are plentiful and in season, freeze them so you can make this salad all year round.

NUTRIENT-RICH BLACK BEAN SOUP
Recipe credit: Chef AJ

(Serves 4-6)

This soup contains over 4 pounds of veggies!!!

<u>Ingredients</u>
6 cups no-sodium broth or water
1 red onion, peeled
3 cans no salt added black beans
4 cloves garlic
1 lb. mushrooms
1 lb. baby bok choy (approx. 3)
1 large sweet potato, peeled if not organic
1 lb. bag frozen corn, defrosted
1½ oz. sundried tomatoes, not oil-packed
1 T cumin
1 T oregano
¼ tsp chipotle powder, or more to taste
¼ to ½ cup lime juice with zest

<u>Preparation</u>
Place water or broth and one bag of the corn in a large soup pot and bring to a boil. Reduce heat and add half of the beans, garlic, sundried tomatoes, onions, sweet potatoes, and greens in a large soup pot. Simmer uncovered for 30 minutes. There is no need to cut anything up as the soup will be blended. If you are using salt-free beans, it is not even necessary to rinse or drain them. Remove from heat and blend soup with an immersion blender.
Stir in cumin, oregano, chipotle paste, lime juice and remaining beans

SWEET POTATO SOUP WITH CANNELLINI BEANS AND RAINBOW CHARD

Recipe credit: Chef AJ, from her book *Unprocessed*

(Serves 4-6)

Ingredients

8 cups water or low-sodium vegetable broth

2 T sundried tomato powder

2 leeks

2-3 large sweet potatoes, peeled and cubed

2 cans cannellini beans, rinsed and drained

1 lb. rainbow chard, chopped

¼ cup fresh-squeezed lemon juice (with zest from lemons)

Preparation

In a large soup pot, bring water to a boil. Reduce heat to medium and add the leeks. Cook for about 10 minutes until soft. Add sweet potatoes and cook another 8-10 minutes until tender. Add the beans and cook for an additional 2 minutes. Remove soup pot from heat and stir in chard so that it wilts. Stir in lemon juice and sun-dried tomato powder. Sprinkle chopped Italian parsley on top, if desired, and garnish with a fresh lemon twist.

Chef's Note: If the ingredients are prepped in advance, it only takes 20 minutes to cook this soup. You can also make this soup with butternut squash or white potatoes in place of sweet potatoes. Swiss chard, collards, spinach, or kale may replace rainbow chard.

CHEF AJ'S DISAPPEARING LASAGNA
Recipe credit: Chef AJ, from her book *Unprocessed*

(Serves 4-6)

Ingredients

2 boxes no-boil rice lasagna noodles (De Boles)

6 cups of your favorite no-oil marinara sauce

1 box, extra-firm water-packed tofu (19 oz.) **OR:**

2 cans (15-oz. each) cannellini beans, drained and rinsed

2 oz. fresh basil leaves

1 cup pine nuts or raw cashews or hemp seeds

2 cloves garlic (or more, to taste)

¼ cup low-sodium miso

¼ cup nutritional yeast

¼ cup lemon juice

1/8 tsp red pepper flakes (or more, to taste)

1 4-oz. can sliced olives, rinsed and drained (optional)

2 lbs. frozen, chopped spinach (defrosted, drained, with all the liquid squeezed out) **OR** 1 lb. frozen kale (defrosted, drained, with all the liquid squeezed out).

2 lbs. sliced mushrooms (crimini or baby bellas preferred)

¼ cup low-sodium tamari

1 large red onion, finely diced

Chef AJ's Faux Parmesan, as garnish (recipe on page XX)

Preparation

Make the filling in a food processor fitted with the "S" blade, by adding the tofu, basil, garlic, lemon juice, miso, pine nuts, red pepper flakes, and nutritional yeast. Puree until smooth. Add drained spinach or kale and process again.

In a large non-stick sauté pan, sauté the onion in 2 tablespoons water until translucent, about 8 minutes, adding more water if necessary. Add garlic, mushrooms, and tamari and sauté until browned. Taste mixture, adding chopped garlic and more tamari according to your taste. Cook until mushrooms appear to be glazed and there is no more liquid left in the pan.

Pour 3 cups of the sauce in a lasagna pan or 9 in. x 13 in. pan. Place one layer of the no-cook noodles on top. Cover the noodles with half of the tofu/spinach mixture, then with half of the mushroom mixture. Place another layer of noodles on the mushroom mixture and add the remaining half of the tofu/spinach mixture and the remaining half of the mushroom mixture. Place one more layer of noodles on top of the mushroom mixture and smother evenly with the remaining 6 cups of sauce. Sprinkle the sliced olives on top of the sauce along with a liberal sprinkling of faux parmesan.

Bake uncovered in a preheated 375° F oven for an hour. Let set 10 minutes before slicing.

Chef's note: If you have time, marinate the sliced mushroom in the tamari several hours in advance or even the night before. Make sure the top layer of noodles is fully covered with sauce.

RED LENTIL SHIITAKE STEW

Recipe credit: Joanna Samorow-Merzer, originally published in *Off the Reservation* by Glen Merzer

(Serves 4)

<u>Ingredients</u>
1 cup dry red lentils
2¼ cups water
4 medium fresh shiitake mushrooms, sliced
1 dry bay leaf
½ cup thinly chopped red onion
½ tsp ginger powder
¾ tsp coriander
½ tsp cumin
2 T chopped fresh parsley for garnish
1 T scallions for garnish
Sea salt, to taste
White pepper, to taste

<u>Preparation</u>
Rinse the red lentils, and soak for at least 20-30 minutes. Discard the soaking water.

In a pot, combine the red lentils with the water and bring to a boil, then simmer for 20 minutes. Add sliced shiitake mushrooms and onion, the bay leaf, ginger powder, coriander, and cumin, and continue simmering for 20 more minutes. In the last minute of simmering, add the sea salt and white pepper and stir in chopped scallions and chopped parsley. Serve with brown rice or mashed potatoes.

BARLEY MISO SOUP

Recipe credit: Joanna Samorow-Merzer, originally published in *Off the Reservation* by Glen Merzer

(Serves 4)

Ingredients

¼ cup dry barley

6 cups plus 5 T water

1 celery stalk, thinly sliced

1 carrot, sliced

2 onions, peeled and diced

½ cup sliced button mushrooms

3 T white miso

2 T chopped parsley

Pinch of sea salt

Toasted nori for garnish (optional)

Preparation

Soak the barley overnight. Discard the soaking water, rinse the barley, and put in a pot with 6 cups of water and pinch of sea salt. Simmer covered until barley is tender, for about 1 hour. Add remaining ingredients except for the parsley. Bring the soup almost to a boil, then lower the flame and simmer, covered, until the vegetables are tender (about 15 minutes).

Prepare the miso: mix the miso paste in a cup with 5 tablespoons of water, then gradually add into it 6-8 tablespoons of the liquid from the soup, and stir well. Remove the soup from the heat and add the miso to it. Bring the soup almost to a boil, lower the flame and simmer for 2-3 minutes. Stir in parsley. Garnish with toasted nori if desired. Serve.

VEGETABLE CASSEROLE

Recipe credit: Joanna Samorow-Merzer, originally published in *Off the Reservation* by Glen Merzer

(Serves 4)

<u>Ingredients</u>
For the casserole batter (wheat or gluten-free):
⅔ cup whole wheat flour or brown rice flour
⅔ cup plus 2 T unsweetened almond milk
2 heaping T unsweetened apple sauce
1¼ tsp baking powder
2 tsp dried marjoram
½ tsp garlic powder
pinch of sea salt

For the filling:
1 small-to-medium yam, sliced
1 small-to-medium Japanese sweet potato, sliced
2 cups fresh sliced button mushrooms (no stems)
½ cup coarsely chopped basil
⅔ cup frozen green peas
½ medium onion, chopped thinly
1 sprig fresh rosemary
1 T chopped fresh sage
½ cup of water
1½ T raw coconut aminos (optional)
Sea salt, to taste
White pepper, to taste (optional)

<u>Preparation</u>

Let the green peas thaw. Steam the sweet potato and yam until soft, then let cool. Cook the mushrooms and onions in ½ cup of water in a sauce pan for about 15-20 minutes; in the last few minutes of cooking add fresh sage. In the last minute of cooking, add sea salt and pepper to taste. You should still have some liquid, which is now an aromatic sauce, in the saucepan.

To make the batter:

Combine all the dry ingredients (flour, baking powder, marjoram, garlic powder, sea salt) and mix well in a bowl. Combine the wet ingredients (almond milk and apple sauce) in a cup. Add the wet mixture to the dry mixture and gently stir to a smooth consistency.

In the casserole dish, begin to create the first layer of the casserole with slices of the steamed Japanese sweet potato. Fill up the empty spaces between the slices with the thawed green peas. Fill in the spaces around the wall of the casserole dish with pieces of fresh rosemary. On the top of the completed first layer, spread a layer of the cooked mushrooms and onions with its liquid. Begin creating the third (and last) layer with slices of the steamed yams. Drizzle over the yams the raw coconut aminos (if using), and scatter the chopped basil. Spread the batter over the top. The spaces between the yam slices will be filled in by the batter.

Pre-heat oven to 350° F. Bake uncovered for 40-50 minutes. Take out of the oven and let stand, covered, for 15 minutes before serving. (The dough doesn't have any oil and to retain moisture it needs to be covered while still hot.) For the gluten-free version, allow to bake for 5-10 extra minutes.

MUNG BEAN CURRY

Recipe credit: Joanna Samorow-Merzer, originally published in *Off the Reservation* by Glen Merzer

(Serves 4-6)

Ingredients

3 cups water
1 cup dried mung beans
2 dry bay leaves
½ medium onion, chopped
3 cloves raw garlic, minced
1 T minced fresh ginger
½ tsp turmeric powder
½ tsp yellow curry
2 T chopped cilantro or sweet basil
1 T freshly squeezed lemon juice
Black pepper, to taste
Sea salt or Bragg's Liquid Aminos, to taste

Preparation

Rinse the mung beans, then soak overnight in water. The following day, discard the water, rinse the beans again, and add 3 cups of water and the bay leaves. Bring the beans almost to a boil, then reduce the flame to simmer. Pick up with a spoon the white foam that forms on the surface of the water and discard. Then simmer covered for about 40 minutes. Add the onions, garlic, ginger, turmeric, and curry, and continue simmering for an additional 20 minutes. When it's done, add pepper to taste, sea salt or Bragg's, lemon juice, chopped cilantro or basil, and stir. Serve over rice.

BUTTERNUT SQUASH AND QUINOA CHILI

Recipe credit: Wendy Solganik of www.HealthyGirlsKitchen.com

(Serves 4-6)

<u>Ingredients</u>

1½ lbs. cubed butternut squash

1 large red or yellow onion, diced

2 15-oz. cans salt-free black beans (or 3 cups of cooked beans)

1 cup uncooked quinoa

1 T minced garlic

3 14.5-oz cans fire-roasted, diced, no-salt-added tomatoes

1 tsp dried jalapeno pepper or 1 jalapeno pepper, deseeded and diced

1½ T salt-free taco seasoning

1 tsp cumin

2 T chili powder

3 T *Benson's Table Tasty* or other salt substitute

1½ cups low-sodium vegetable broth, plus at least 1 more cup for desired consistency

3 cups frozen corn kernels

Optional garnishes: scallions, cilantro

<u>Preparation</u>

Place 1½ cups of the vegetable broth and all other ingredients except for the corn into an *Instant Pot* electric pressure cooker and stir. Cook on high pressure for 15 minutes. You can do quick or natural release, it doesn't matter. Once cooked, add corn and stir. Add as much or as little additional vegetable broth to achieve the desired consistency for your palate. It's great really thick and yummy without added broth, but nice also with a more stew-like consistency.

HGK's RATATOUILLE

Recipe credit: Wendy Solganik (www.HealthyGirlsKitchen.com)
(Serves a Crowd)

Ingredients
1 large eggplant, cut into 1 in. cubes (approximately 9 cups)
Vegetable broth, for sautéing
1 very large onion, diced (approximately 4 cups)
8 cloves garlic, minced (2 heaping T)
2 cups medium dice carrots
1 very large red pepper, medium dice (or orange or yellow, approximately 3 cups)
6 cups chopped tomatoes
1 can tomato paste
1 tsp dried thyme
1 T dried basil
1 T parsley
1 large zucchini, cut into 1" cubes (approx. 6 cups)
1 medium yellow squash, cut into 1" cubes (approx. 4 cups)
Salt, to taste (optional)
½ - 1 tsp ground pepper

Preparation
Preheat the oven to 375° F.
Place cubed eggplant on a parchment paper lined baking sheet (it's okay if cubes are piled on each other) and bake for 30 minutes. Place a large Dutch oven or soup pot over medium high heat. Line the base of the pot with vegetable broth. When broth is boiling, add onion and cook, stirring occasionally, for 5 minutes.

Lower heat to prevent burning if necessary. Add garlic and stir. Cook for 3 minutes, watching heat to prevent burning. Add carrots and stir. Cook for 10 minutes. Add broth and adjust heat if necessary to prevent burning. Add red pepper, tomatoes, tomato paste, thyme, basil and parsley and stir.

Return heat to medium and cook for 8 minutes. The stew should come to a simmer and not a boil. Add zucchini and yellow squash and stir. Cook for 10 minutes, stirring occasionally. Add roasted eggplant cubes and stir. Taste and add salt (optional) and pepper. Let simmer, partially covered, for 30 minutes.

Serve alone, over baked potatoes, whole wheat couscous, pasta or warm polenta. Can be served cold, warm or hot.

CRISPY CREAMY TWICE BAKED BROCCOLI AND CHEEZE POTATOES

Recipe credit: Wendy Solganik of www.HealthyGirlsKitchen.com
(Serves 6)

Chef's Note: There are five steps to this process. The first two steps can be done well in advance. I baked the potatoes in the morning before I left for work and then refrigerated the baked potatoes until I got home. I prepared the cheezy sauce days in advance.

Bake the Potatoes
Ingredients
6 medium russet potatoes

Preparation
Preheat oven to 350° F and position rack in middle. Wash potatoes thoroughly with cold running water. Dry, then using a standard fork poke 8 to 12 deep holes all over the spud so that moisture can escape during cooking. Place potatoes directly on rack in middle of oven. (Optional: place a baking sheet on the lower rack to catch any drippings.)
Bake 1 hour and 15 minutes or until skin feels crisp but flesh beneath feels soft. Carefully remove from oven and set aside to cool.
NOTE: If you're cooking less than 6 potatoes, you might need to decrease the cooking time by up to 15 minutes.
Steam the broccoli to desired softness, keeping in mind it will cook some more.

Prepare the Cheezy Sauce
Ingredients
1 15-oz. can chickpeas, rinsed and drained (1½ cups cooked chickpeas)
2 T + 1 tsp nutritional yeast

1½ T tahini
1½ T white wine vinegar
1 T + 1 tsp light miso paste
1 tsp onion powder
½ tsp paprika
½ tsp turmeric
¼ tsp garlic powder
¼ tsp dry mustard
½ tsp salt (optional)
½ cup alternative milk, (unsweetened almond milk recommended)

Steam the broccoli
Ingredients
3 cups chopped broccoli
Steam to desired softness, keeping in mind it will cook some more.

Place all ingredients into the bowl of a food processor fitted with the "S" blade. Process until mixture is smooth, scraping down sides as necessary.

Assemble the potatoes:
Preheat oven to 400° F. Prepare a baking tray by lining it with parchment paper.

When the potatoes are cool, slice each one in half lengthwise. Scoop out the flesh of each half and place it into a large bowl. Reserve the potato skins.

When all of the flesh is in the bowl, place the cheezy sauce into the bowl and mash with a potato masher until well incorporated.
Place 2 cups of the steamed and chopped broccoli into the bowl and stir well.

Using a soup spoon, scoop the potato/broccoli mixture back into the potato skins. Tamp mixture down into the skin (you can use your fingers during the process) and fill until the mixture is piled high into the potato skin. Place on prepared baking tray and repeat until all skins are stuffed. Top off each potato half with some of the remaining cup of chopped broccoli. Smush the broccoli into the potato mixture.

Bake the stuffed potatoes for 20 minutes.

Turn heat on oven to broil. Let potatoes and broccoli crisp for a few minutes under the broiler, watching that the potatoes do not get too burned. Serve immediately.

Chef's Note: Refrigerates well, so makes excellent leftovers. These would be great to prepare in advance and reheat any time you are having company or bringing food over to someone else's home.

QUINNY'S SRI LANKAN KALE with BLACK BEANS and SWEET POTATOES

Recipe credit: Wendy Solganik of www.HealthyGirlsKitchen.com

(Serves 2)

Ingredients

1 med. (red or white or yellow) onion, chopped

1-2 hot chili peppers, seeded and chopped or hot chili flakes to taste

12 oz. kale (or other greens), stems removed and thinly sliced

2 med.-large sweet potatoes, cut into approximately 1 in. cubes

¼ tsp ground cumin

Grated black pepper, to taste

½ cup shredded coconut (the partially defatted version is recommended)

1 can black beans, drained and rinsed

Juice of 1 lime

Salt, to taste

Preparation

In low sodium vegetable broth or water, sauté onions and chili peppers/ chili pepper flakes until soft. Add cumin and stir.

Add sweet potatoes and cook, stirring frequently, on medium to high heat until the potatoes begin to soften some, but not turn to mush, approximately 10 minutes.

Add kale and splash of broth, along with black pepper. Cover and cook, stirring occasionally, until kale is wilted but bright green, approximately 5 minutes.

Add coconut, black beans, lime juice and about 1/4 cup of vegetable broth if mix is dry. Heat through. Add salt to taste. Serve immediately and wish you had made more.

CUBAN BLACK BEANS WITH KALE

Recipe credit: Wendy Solganik of www.HealthyGirlsKitchen.com

(Serves 4 as a main dish, 8 as a side dish)

Ingredients

Low sodium vegetable broth, a few T

1 large yellow onion, diced

4 garlic cloves, minced

1 T grated fresh ginger (using a microplaner if you have one)

2 tsp chili powder

1 tsp cumin

½ tsp paprika

½ tsp cinnamon

2 15-oz. cans black beans, undrained

4 cups finely chopped kale or other greens

2 T fresh lemon or lime juice (whatever you have on hand)

Optional: hot sauce, to taste

Preparation

Place a medium pot over medium-high heat and coat the bottom of the pot with low sodium vegetable broth. When broth is boiling add onion and stir. Cook for 5 minutes, stirring frequently.

Lower heat to medium. Add garlic and ginger. Cook until onions are translucent, stirring frequently and adding more broth if necessary to prevent burning.

Add chili powder, cumin, paprika and cinnamon. Stir.

Add undrained black beans and stir. Mash with the back of a fork or a potato masher, leaving some of the beans whole.

Add kale and stir. Lower heat to low and let simmer until mixture thickens. Stir in lime or lemon juice and hot sauce (optional) to taste. Cover until ready to serve.

EASY ALOO GOBI WITH KALE

Recipe credit: Wendy Solganik of www.HealthyGirlsKitchen.com
(Serves 4)

Ingredients

3 T or more vegetable broth for sautéing
1 bag frozen chopped onions (or 1 medium yellow onion, chopped)
1 T curry powder
1 T cumin
1 28-oz. can diced tomatoes (low sodium and/or fire roasted optional)
3 cups medium dice new potatoes
½ can light coconut milk or ¾ cups plant-based milk plus 1/2 tsp coconut extract
1 10-oz. bag frozen cauliflower, or 1/2 small-medium head cauliflower cut into large bite-sized pieces
1 15-oz. can chickpeas, drained and rinsed or 1 ½ cups cooked chickpeas
Destemmed, rough-chopped kale, as much as you would like
Salt, to taste (optional)
Fresh cilantro, for garnish

Preparation

Place a large pot over medium-high heat and add vegetable broth. When broth is bubbling, add onions and stir. "Sauté" onions until they are translucent and soft, at least 10 minutes, lowering the heat as is necessary to prevent burning.

Add curry powder and cumin and stir. Let cook for 2 minutes, adding a bit more broth if necessary to prevent sticking.

Add diced tomatoes, potatoes, and coconut milk (or a lower-fat plant milk with a splash of coconut extract) stir and bring to a boil. Turn heat to low and let simmer for 20 minutes.

Add cauliflower and stir. Simmer for 10 minutes.

Add chickpeas and stir.

Add as much chopped kale as you would like and stir. Let simmer until kale has wilted and potatoes are soft. Serve garnished with cilantro.

ITALIAN WHITE BEAN, KALE, AND POTATO STEW

Recipe credit: **Wendy Solganik of** www.HealthyGirlsKitchen.com

(Serves 6)

Ingredients

1 cup diced red or white onion

3 cloves garlic

2 28-oz. cans diced tomatoes (salt-free if you prefer)

¼-½ tsp red pepper flakes

5 cups medium dice red skinned potatoes (any boiling potato will do)

1 T dried oregano

1 T dried parsley

6-8 packed cups of kale, after it has been destemmed and chopped

2 15-oz. cans cannellini beans, drained and rinsed

Salt (optional)

Preparation

Place a large soup/stock pot over a medium-high flame and pour some of the liquid from one of the cans of the diced tomatoes into the pot to cover the base of the pot. When the tomato liquid starts to bubble, add the onion and stir. Lower heat a little. Press garlic into pot. Add red pepper flakes (to taste). Continue to cook and stir, lowering heat as the time passes, for a total of about 10 minutes or until onions are soft.

Add the rest of the first can of diced tomatoes and the entire second can into the pot. Bring heat up to medium-high again so that tomatoes begin to simmer. Place diced potatoes, oregano and parsley into the pot and stir. Cover pot, lower heat to low and simmer for 20 minutes.

Place all of the kale into the pot and cover the pot again. Let kale steam and shrink for 3 minutes. Uncover pot and stir in kale. Add cannellini beans and stir. Taste and season with salt (optional). If potatoes are not as soft as you desire, continue to let simmer until potatoes reach desired doneness.

MUSHROOM, KALE, AND SPINACH ENCHILADA CASSEROLE WITH SALSA VERDE AND ROASTED POBLANO CREAM

Recipe credit: Wendy Solganik of www.HealthyGirlsKitchen.com

(Serves 8)

Ingredients

1 batch Mushroom, Kale and Spinach Filling (see recipe below)

7-9 corn or medium-sized 100% whole wheat tortillas

2 12-oz. jars salsa verde (low sodium if you can find it)

1 recipe Roasted Poblano Cream (see recipe below)

Diced red onion

Chopped cilantro

Fresh lime

Ingredients for the Mushroom, Kale and Spinach Filling:

Low sodium vegetable broth for sautéing

1½ cups chopped red onion

2 garlic cloves, minced

12-16 oz. sliced mushrooms

6 packed cups kale, either baby kale or regular kale that has been destemmed before rough chopping

3 cups packed spinach

1½ cups frozen corn kernels, fire-roasted optional

1 15-oz. can black beans, rinsed and drained

Preparation

Preheat oven to 350° F.

Place a large skillet over high heat. Coat the base of the skillet with vegetable broth. When broth is simmering, add onions and stir. Let onions sauté, stirring frequently, until onions are translucent. You will need turn the heat down as the onions cook to prevent burning.

Add garlic and stir. Let cook for 5 minutes. Add mushrooms and stir. Let cook, stirring occasionally, for 10 minutes or until they cook down. Add kale and stir. Cook for 7 minutes or until kale has wilted. Add spinach and stir. Cook for 5 minutes or until spinach has wilted.

Add ½ jar of salsa verde and stir. Add frozen corn and black beans. Remove from heat.

<u>Ingredients for the Roasted Poblano Cream</u>
1 poblano pepper
¾ cup raw unsalted cashews (soaked for 30 minutes, if you think of it)
6 T water
1 small garlic clove
2 T minced red onion
2 T fresh lemon juice
salt, to taste (about ½ teaspoon)

Roast the poblano pepper. You can do this in one of two ways:
(1) Place under the broiler for 20 or so minutes, until blistered on all sides (time will vary depending on the heat of your broiler). When it's fully blistered, remove and place in a bowl and cover (not touching) with plastic wrap or at towel. Set aside for 15 minutes or so, until it's cool enough to handle. Using your fingers, slide off the skin and remove the stem and seeds. Or:
(2) Place poblano pepper directly on top of a gas flame. Turn frequently until pepper is blackened on all sides. Follow directions above from placing pepper in a bowl and covering.

Blend roasted poblano and all ingredients in a high-powered blender (best results from a Vitamix or similar) or food processor. Taste and adjust seasonings to your liking. Set aside.

To assemble the enchiladas:
Begin by coating the base of a 9 in. by 13 in. casserole with 1/3 jar of salsa verde. Place tortillas in a single layer to cover the bottom of the casserole, cutting one tortilla into pieces to fill in large gaps.
Scoop half of the Mushroom, Kale and Spinach filling over the tortillas and gently smooth out into one uniform layer. Repeat with another layer of tortillas. Pour 1/3 of the jar of salsa verde over the tortillas and spread evenly over tortillas.

Scoop other half of Mushroom, Kale and Spinach filling over tortillas, smoothing filling into a uniform layer. Place another layer of tortillas followed by the final 1/3 of the jar of salsa verde spread over the tortillas.

Bake at 350° F for 30 minutes.

Serve with a dollop of Roasted Poblano Cream and a generous amount of diced red onion and chopped cilantro. Squeeze some fresh lime juice over the top.

HGK's ALOO BAINGAN (POTATO AND EGGPLANT)

Recipe credit: Wendy Solganik of www.HealthyGirlsKitchen.com
Inspired by a recipe from Manjula's Kitchen
(Serves 3-4)

Ingredients
1 medium purple eggplant, unpeeled, cut into ½ in. cubes
5 medium boiling potatoes, peeled and cut into ½ in. cubes
1 medium tomato cut into ½ in. cubes
1½ cups fat-free tomato sauce (I have been really into the Muir Glen brand lately—check the labels for the varieties with no fat)
Cooking spray
Pinch of asafoetida (hing) (don't stress out if you don't have this ingredient, just leave it out)
1 tsp cumin seed
1 small chopped green chili (jalapeno-deseeded), adjust to taste!
1 tsp grated ginger
1 T coriander powder
½ tsp turmeric
½ tsp paprika
1 tsp salt, adjust to taste
2 T or more chopped cilantro

Preparation
Preheat your oven to 400° F and line two cookie sheets with aluminum foil. Spray foil lightly with cooking spray and lay out chopped eggplant pieces on one sheet and chopped potato pieces on the other. Roast eggplant for approximately 15 minutes, until it is starting to soften, but not turn into mush. Roast potato for approximately 25 minutes until edges of potato pieces are starting to brown and potato is just cooked.

While eggplant and potato are roasting, in a small bowl, mix the grated ginger, jalapeno pepper, coriander powder, paprika, turmeric, and 2 tablespoons of water to make a paste.

Spray the base of a pot with cooking spray and heat the pot over medium heat. Test the heat by adding one cumin seed to the pot; if seed cracks right away pot is heated to the right temperature.

Add cumin seeds and asafetida, if using, after seeds crack. Add the spice mixture and stir-fry for 20 seconds, stirring continuously.

Add chopped tomato and stir-fry for a minute. Add tomato sauce.

Add roasted potatoes and eggplant. Mix it gently, let it simmer for three to four minutes on medium-low heat. Turn off the heat and add chopped cilantro. Mix it well.

QUINOA CURRY BOWL
Recipe credit: Cathy Fisher
(Serves 2 as main dish, 4 as side dish)

Ingredients
1½ cups water
¾ cup quinoa (dry)
1 tsp granulated onion
½ tsp curry powder
1 bag (16 oz.) frozen "stir fry" blend vegetables
1 T minced garlic (4 to 5 medium cloves)
1 tsp minced fresh ginger
1 tsp curry powder
2 T tahini (ground sesame paste)
½ avocado (optional)
Sesame seeds to garnish (optional)

Preparation
Stir the water, quinoa, granulated onion, and ½ teaspoon curry powder together in a medium saucepan, and bring to a boil. Reduce heat to a low simmer and cook covered with a tight-fitting lid for 15 minutes.

While the quinoa is cooking, place the frozen vegetables into a skillet or soup pot on medium-low heat covered so the vegetables can thaw and soften. Stir occasionally, adding a little water if needed. While the vegetables are warming, mince the garlic and ginger.

When the vegetables have thawed and softened (5 to 10 minutes), increase the heat to medium-high and stir in the garlic, ginger, and 1 tea-spoon curry powder; l cook stirring for 1 to 2 minutes. Remove the pan from the heat and add the tahini, adding a little water as needed to mix thoroughly. Stir the quinoa into the vegetables. Serve as is or with diced avocado and/or sesame seeds on top.

MUSHROOM-BASIL AU GRATIN
Recipe credit: Cathy Fisher
(Serves 6-8)

<u>Ingredients</u>
4-5 large Yukon potatoes, sliced thinly
8 large white or crimini mushrooms, sliced thinly
1 yellow onion, sliced thinly
1 bunch chard
½ bunch fresh basil (about 20 leaves)

Sauce:
1/3 cup raw cashews
1 cup water
½ cup soy milk
½ cup parsley leaves
2 green onions, diced
½ tsp garlic powder

<u>Preparation</u>
In a high-speed blender, grind the cashews by themselves first until fine; add the water, soy milk, parsley, green onions and garlic powder, and blend thoroughly. Set aside.

To prepare the vegetables, using a mandolin slicer with the thin slicing blade (as if you were making potato chips), slice the potatoes, mushrooms and onion, and set aside in separate bowls. Remove the thickest stems from the chard leaves, and remove the leaves of basil from their stems; wash both and set aside.

In a 13 in. x9 in. rectangular glass baking dish, layer vegetables in this order, starting with a thin layer of sauce in the bottom of the dish (you do not need to oil the pan): potatoes, mushrooms, onions, basil, chard, sauce. Add a second layer of vegetables and sauce, then finish with a final layer of potatoes, pouring the last bit of sauce over the top of them. Cover with aluminum foil and bake at 400° F for 35 minutes. Remove the foil and cook an additional 15 minutes until lightly browned on top (optional: grind some cashews on top first). Remove and let sit for at least 5 minutes before serving.

HOPPIN' JOHN WITH AVOCADO-CUCUMBER DRESSING
Recipe Credit: Cathy Fisher
(Serves 4)

<u>Ingredients</u>
1 medium onion or shallot, chopped
1 bell pepper, seeded and diced
2 ribs celery or 1 fennel bulb, diced
1 to 2 cloves garlic, minced
½ tsp dried thyme
½ tsp dried basil
½ tsp cumin
2 cans black-eyed peas (1½ cups), rinsed
2 green onions, chopped
½ cup parsley, chopped
6 leaves collard greens, chopped
Cooked brown rice for 4

<u>Preparation</u>
Using water as needed, sauté the onion, bell pepper, celery or fennel on medium-high for a few minutes until soft. Add the garlic, thyme, basil and cumin and sauté another minute.
Mix in the black-eyed peas, green onions, parsley and collard greens, and cook until the collards are softened. Serve as is topped with the Avocado-Cucumber dressing (below) over brown rice.

Avocado-Cucumber Dressing
⅔ cup water
2 tsp lemon juice or apple cider vinegar
1 avocado, diced

½ tsp garlic powder
½ cucumber (with seeds), diced
½ cup raw spinach, chopped
1 green onion, chopped

Combine all ingredients in a blender until smooth. Add water as needed.

TOMATO RICE SOUP
Recipe credit: Cathy Fisher

(Serves 6-8)

<u>INGREDIENTS</u>

1 medium yellow or white onion, chopped (2 cups)

6½ cups water

1 can (15 oz.) Navy or white beans, drained and rinsed (or 1½ cups)

¾ cup uncooked, long-grain brown rice

2 cans (14.5 oz. each) diced tomatoes

2 ribs celery, chopped

5 medium cremini or white mushrooms, sliced (about 2 cups)

1 T dried Italian herb blend

1½ tsp granulated garlic

4 leaves Swiss chard (or other greens), coarsely chopped (2 to 3 cups)

15 large leaves fresh basil, chopped (about 1 cup)

<u>Preparation</u>

Place 1 tablespoon of water into a soup pot on high heat. When the water begins to sputter, add the onion and cook stirring for 3 to 5 minutes, until the onions become softened.

Add the water, beans, rice, diced tomatoes (including juice), celery, mushrooms, dried Italian herbs, and granulated garlic, and stir. Bring to a boil, and then reduce heat to a simmer. Cover and cook for 25 minutes. Stir in the chard and cook covered for 10 more minutes. Stir in the basil and serve.

QUINOA-POLENTA & BBQ SAUCE
Recipe credit: Cathy Fisher
(Serves 4-6)

<u>Ingredients</u>
2½ cups water
½ cup organic medium- or coarse-grind cornmeal
½ cup uncooked (dry) quinoa
2 tsp granulated garlic
1½ tsp granulated onion
1½ tsp dried oregano (or Mexican spice blend)
1 tsp chili powder

<u>Preparation</u>
Place all ingredients into a saucepan, and on high heat bring to a boil, stirring frequently. Reduce heat to a low simmer and cook for 20 minutes covered, stirring 2 or 3 times during (replacing the lid each time).
When done simmering, the batter should be very thick. Spread into an 8 in. ×8 in. square pan lined with parchment paper. Cook at 400° F for 15-20 minutes, until the top crust is deeper in color but not browned (see photo below). Cut into 4-6 pieces.

BBQ Sauce:
<u>Ingredients</u>
1-1/2 cups water
1 can (6-oz.) tomato paste
½ cup black beans (drained, rinsed)
¼ cup brown raisins
2 T stone-ground mustard
1 tsp chili powder
1 tsp apple cider or brown rice vinegar

¾ tsp granulated garlic
¾ tsp granulated onion

<u>Directions</u>
Place all ingredients into a blender and blend for 1-2 minutes, until smooth. Pour into a saucepan.

On medium heat, bring to just almost boiling then reduce to a low simmer and cook for 15 minutes, stirring occasionally. Serve hot or cold.

BIBIMBAP
Recipe Credit: Del Sroufe
(Serves 4)

Ingredients
4 cups cooked brown rice
1 recipe Simple Candied Sweet Potatoes
4 cups fresh spinach, steamed until wilted, about 4 to 5 minutes
2 cups mung bean sprouts
2 carrots, grated
Gochujang sauce, to taste

To serve, divide the rice between four bowls and arrange the vegetables around and over the rice. Let each person add gochujang sauce to taste. Each person mixes everything in their bowl together and enjoys!

SIMPLE CANDIED SWEET POTATOES
Serves 4

Ingredients
3 cups sweet potatoes, peeled and diced into 1/2-inch cubes
¾ cup Best Date Syrup Ever
Black sesame seeds (garnish)

Preparation
Steam the sweet potatoes for 8 to 10 minutes, until tender. While they steam, add the date syrup to a large skillet with 1 /4 cup water and bring it to a boil. Let it simmer for 5 minutes. Add the steamed sweet potatoes and let them cook for another minute. Serve garnished with the black sesame seeds.

BEST DATE SYRUP EVER
Makes 3 Cups

<u>Ingredients</u>
2 cups pitted Medjool dates
½ tsp Stevia powder
1 ½ - 2 cups water

<u>Preparation</u>
Place all ingredients in a blender and puree until smooth and creamy. Add water as needed to get the mixture to blend. Store refrigerated for up to one week.

CREAMY PASTA AND BROCCOLI
Recipe Credit: Del Sroufe
(Serves 4)

<u>Ingredients</u>
12 oz. whole-grain penne pasta
1 head broccoli, cut into florets
2 large leeks, thinly sliced
½ cup white wine
2 cups Cauliflower Purée
2 T nutritional yeast
2 tsp Dijon mustard
Zest of 1 lemon
Pinch of ground nutmeg
Sea salt and black pepper to taste

<u>Preparation</u>
Cook the pasta according to package instructions. Add the broccoli to the pot of pasta in the last 4 minutes of cooking. While the pasta and broccoli cook, sauté the leeks in a large skillet until they are tender, about 7 to 8 minutes. Add water 1 to 2 tablespoons at a time to keep the leeks from sticking. Turn the heat up to high, add the wine, and cook until the liquid is reduced by half. Add the cauliflower purée, nutritional yeast, Dijon mustard, lemon zest, and nutmeg. Add salt and pepper to taste.

While the sauce is reducing, drain the cooked pasta and broccoli. Before serving, toss with the sauce.

CAULIFLOWER PUREE
Makes 2 Cups

Ingredients
3 cups cauliflower florets
¾ to 1 cup water or vegetable stock
Sea salt to taste

Preparation
Place the cauliflower in a steamer and cook until very tender, about 8 to
10 minutes. Place the florets in a blender and puree with enough water
to make a creamy consistency. Season with salt or salt substitute.

CREOLE CORN CHOWDER
Recipe Credit: Del Sroufe
(Serves 6)

Ingredients
1 large yellow onion, diced
1 stalk celery, diced
1 large red bell pepper, diced
4 ears corn, kernels removed from the cobs (about 3 cups)
1 T Creole Spice Blend, or use more or less to taste (store-bought, or recipe follows)
1 bay leaf
2 cups vegetable stock
1 large russet potato, peeled and diced
2 cups Cauliflower Purée (recipe above)
2 T nutritional yeast
Sea salt and black pepper to taste

Preparation
Sauté the onion, celery, and red bell pepper in a large saucepan over medium heat for 7 to 8 minutes. Add water 1 to 2 tablespoons at a time to keep the vegetables from sticking. Add the corn and Creole Spice Blend, and cook for another minute.

Add the bay leaf, vegetable stock, and diced potato, and cook, covered, over medium-low heat for 20 minutes, until the potatoes are tender. Add the cauliflower purée, nutritional yeast, and sea salt and pepper to taste, and cook over medium-low heat for another 10 minutes.

CREOLE SPICE BLEND

Ingredients

2 T sweet paprika

1 T dried oregano

1 T dried basil

1 T granulated onion

1 T granulated garlic

2 tsp dried thyme

2 tsp cayenne pepper, or use more or less to taste

2 tsp white pepper, or use more or less to taste

1 tsp black pepper

Preparation

Combine everything in a small bowl and mix well. Store in an airtight container for up to three months.

DEL'S BIG BREAKFAST CASSEROLE
Recipe Credit: Del Sroufe
(Serves 6 to 8)

Ingredients
4 medium red-skin potatoes, scrubbed and thinly sliced
3 large yellow onions, thinly sliced
1 pound firm tofu
1 12-oz. package extra-firm silken tofu
2 medium yellow onions, diced
1 red bell pepper, diced
1 8-oz. package sliced button mushrooms
1 10-oz. package frozen broccoli, thawed
4 cloves garlic, minced
1 T dried basil
1 tsp dried sage
½ tsp ground fennel seeds
1 tsp crushed red pepper
6 T nutritional yeast
Sea salt to taste
½ tsp black pepper

Preheat the oven to 350° F. Steam the potatoes for 6 to 8 minutes, until tender but still firm. While the potatoes steam, sauté the three large onions in a medium skillet until caramelized, about 12 minutes. Add water 1 to 2 tablespoons at a time to keep them from sticking. Set them aside. Place the firm tofu and silken tofu in a large bowl and mash to the consistency of ricotta cheese. Set it aside.

Heat a large skillet over medium-high heat, add the diced medium onions, red bell peppers, mushrooms, and broccoli, and sauté for 5 to

6 minutes, until the vegetables are tender. Add the garlic, basil, sage, fennel, and crushed red pepper, and cook for another minute. Add the onion mixture to the tofu along with the nutritional yeast, salt, and pepper. Mix well. Press the tofu filling into a 9 in. ×13 in. nonstick baking dish. Top with the steamed potatoes and then the caramelized onions. Bake for 45 minutes.

FALAFEL BOWL
Recipe Credit: Del Sroufe
(Serves 4)

Ingredients
4 cups cooked brown rice
1 package frozen mixed vegetables, cooked according to package instructions
1 recipe Falafel (follows)
1 cup Green Sauce (follows)
Chopped green onion or cilantro, for garnish

Preparation
Put 1 cup of cooked brown rice in the bottom of each of the four bowls. Top each bowl with some of the cooked vegetables, Falafel, and Green Sauce. Garnish with chopped green onion, cilantro, or both.

GREEN SAUCE
Makes 1 ¾ Cups

Ingredients
1 12-oz. package Mori-Nu Silken Lite Firm Tofu
¾ cup chopped fresh cilantro
¼ cup tahini (not raw)
2 T lemon juice
4 cloves garlic
2 tsp sea salt
¼ tsp cayenne pepper

Preparation
Combine all ingredients in a blender and puree until smooth and creamy.
Store refrigerated in an airtight container for up to 7 days.

Tip
If you leave out the tahini to decrease the fat content, increase the cilantro to 1 cup.

FALAFEL
Makes 4 Servings

Ingredients
2 15-oz. cans garbanzo beans (chickpeas), drained and rinsed
1 medium yellow onion, chopped
6 cloves garlic, chopped
4 T fresh parsley, chopped
1 T arrowroot powder
4 tsp ground coriander
2 tsp ground cumin
Sea salt and black pepper to taste

Preparation
Preheat the oven to 375° F. Add everything to a food processor and process, leaving a little texture to the beans. Using a small ice cream scoop or tablespoon, shape the mixture into balls. Place on a nonstick baking sheet and bake for 10 minutes. Turn the falafel over and bake for another 8–10 minutes.

BUDDHA BOWL

Recipe Credit: Kim Campbell, *The PlantPure Nation Cookbook*

(Serves 4)

Ingredients

1 cup quinoa

2 cups water

1 cup broccoli, cut into florets

1 ½ cups chopped dinosaur kale

3 green onions, sliced

½ carrot, shredded

1 avocado, pitted and diced

½ red bell pepper, seeded and diced

½ cup halved cherry tomatoes

1 cup canned chickpeas, rinsed and drained

½ cup Sweet Tahini Dressing (follows)

Preparation

Rinse the quinoa, which can have a bitter taste if not rinsed thoroughly. Add the quinoa and the water to a pot, bring to a boil over medium-high heat, then reduce the heat to a simmer. Cover and cook until all the liquid is absorbed. Lightly steam the broccoli and kale in a small amount of water until the colors are bright green.

Add the green onions, carrot, avocado, bell pepper, tomatoes, and chickpeas to a large mixing bowl along with the steamed kale and broccoli. Toss to combine. Assemble the Buddha bowl by placing warm cooked quinoa in a bowl and tossing with veggies and chickpeas. Drizzle the tahini dressing over the top and serve.

SWEET TAHINI DRESSING
Serves 4-6

Ingredients
¼ cup tahini
¼ cup water
1 T maple syrup
¼ cup balsamic vinegar
3 T lemon juice
2 garlic cloves, minced
2 tablespoons chopped fresh
Parsley
1 tsp white miso paste
½ tsp sea salt

Preparation
Place all the ingredients in a blender and process until smooth.

CHICKPEA-CRANBERRY SALAD
Recipe Credit: Kim Campbell, *The PlantPure Nation Cookbook*
(Serves 6)

Ingredients
¼ cup tahini
¼ cup rice vinegar
¼ cup water
2 T agave nectar
½ tsp dried dill weed
¼ tsp red pepper flakes
Two 15-oz. cans chickpeas, rinsed and drained
½ cup diced celery
1 carrot, diced small or shredded
½ cup dried cranberries
½ cup finely chopped walnuts
½ cup diced red onion
¼ cup chopped fresh parsley
¼ tsp sea salt
¼ tsp black pepper

Preparation
Start by mixing the dressing. In a small bowl, combine the tahini, vinegar, water, agave, dill, and red pepper flakes. Set aside so the flavors come together. You can play with the flavor of vinegar you like. Rice vinegar is a good option because it's mild. In a medium to large bowl, add the chickpeas and roughly mash with a strong fork or potato masher. Add the celery, carrot, cranberries, nuts, red onion, parsley, salt, pepper, and tahini dressing. Mix well. Serve at room temperature or let chill in the refrigerator for an hour before serving.

CRUNCHY CHICKPEA TACOS
Recipe Credit: Kim Campbell, *The PlantPure Nation Cookbook*
(Serves 6 tacos)

Ingredients
6 corn or flour tortillas
One 15-oz. can chickpeas, rinsed and drained
½ tsp ancho chili powder
3 cups shredded green cabbage
1 cup shredded carrot
½ cup thinly sliced red onion
½ cup seeded and small diced poblano pepper
½ cup sliced green onion
¼ cup chopped fresh cilantro
¼ cup Tofu Cashew Mayonnaise (follows)
2 T lime juice
¼ tsp sea salt
1 avocado, pitted and sliced
1 T Sriracha (optional)

Preparation
Preheat the oven to 375°F. Shape the tortillas by placing them in a non-stick oven-safe bowl and baking them in the oven until crispy, 5–10 minutes. In a large mixing bowl, smash the chickpeas with a fork and sprinkle with the chili powder. Add the cabbage, carrot, red onion, poblano pepper, green onion, cilantro, mayonnaise, and lime juice. Mix thoroughly, adding salt last. Divide the salad mixture among the taco bowls and top with the sliced avocado. Add Sriracha if you like your tacos spicy.

TOFU CASHEW MAYONNAISE
Makes 2 Cups

Ingredients

¼ cup raw cashews, soaked in water to cover for 2–3 hours, then drained

7 oz. extra-firm tofu

½ tsp sea salt

½ tsp tahini

4 tsp lemon juice

1 ½ tsp white vinegar

1 T Dijon mustard

2 T apple cider vinegar

2 ½ tsp agave nectar

2 T water

¼ tsp xanthan gum

Preparation

Soaking the cashews in water for a few hours will reduce blending time. If you are not using a Vitamix, I highly recommend soaking the cashews so they blend into a smooth and creamy texture. Place all the ingredients in a Vitamix or other high-powered blender. Blend until smooth and shiny.

EDAMAME BURGERS

Recipe Credit: Kim Campbell, *The PlantPure Nation Cookbook*

(Serves 6 Burgers)

Ingredients

4 cups frozen shelled edamame, cooked

2 cups frozen mixed vegetable stir-fry blend, thawed

1 T flax meal

2 T hot water

¼ cup orange juice

¼ tsp low-sodium soy sauce

1 T agave nectar

¼ tsp Dijon mustard

1 cup whole wheat bread crumbs

½ tsp sea salt

¼ tsp black pepper

1 tsp lemon juice

6 whole wheat burger buns

6 green-leaf lettuce leaves

1 ½ cups sprouts

¾ cup Cilantro-Wasabi Aioli (follows)

Preparation

Preheat oven to 375°F. Line a baking sheet with parchment paper and set aside. Place the cooked edamame and thawed stir-fry blend into a food processor. Pulse multiple times until the ingredients are well blended. It should be green and have a fine consistency similar to that of short-grain rice. In a small bowl, combine the flax meal and water. Allow to sit for 2–3 minutes. Remove the vegetable mixture from the food processor and place in a large mixing bowl. Add the flax mixture and fold together. Add the orange juice, soy sauce, agave, Dijon mustard, breadcrumbs, salt, pepper, and lemon juice to the vegetables and mix well. Form into 6 patties and place on the prepared baking sheet. Bake for 10–15 minutes. Flip and continue baking for an additional 10–15 minutes. Remove from the oven and allow the burgers to set for about 5 minutes before serving. Serve on a whole-wheat bun topped with lettuce, sprouts, and Cilantro-Wasabi Aioli.

CILANTRO-WASABI AIOLI

Serves 8

Ingredients
¼ cup raw cashews, soaked in water to cover for 2–3 hours, then drained
¼ cup water
¼ cup silken tofu
1 clove garlic
1 tsp wasabi paste
1 tsp low-sodium soy sauce
½ tsp lemon juice
1 tsp pureed ginger
1 T apple cider vinegar
1 T chopped fresh cilantro
½ tsp sea salt

Preparation
Soaking the cashews in water for a few hours will reduce blending time. If you are not using a Vitamix, soak the cashews so they blend into a smooth and creamy texture. Combine all the ingredients in a Vitamix or other high-powered blender and process on high speed until smooth and creamy. Remove from the blender and chill to thicken. Serve chilled.

SPINACH AND BROCCOLI ENCHILADAS

Recipe Credit: Kim Campbell, *The PlantPure Nation Cookbook*

(Serves 4-6 Enchiladas)

<u>Ingredients</u>

10 oz. chopped frozen spinach

1 onion, diced

12 oz. broccoli, chopped

½ cup water

3 cups salsa (medium heat), divided

1 tsp garlic powder

1 tsp Mrs. Dash Southwest Chipotle Seasoning Blend or Mexican Spice Blend

8 oz. extra-firm tofu, drained and crumbled

2 T nutritional yeast flakes

2 T tahini

4–6 large whole wheat tortillas

<u>Preparation</u>

Preheat oven to 350°F. Thaw and drain the frozen spinach. In a large skillet over medium heat, sauté the onion, spinach, and chopped broccoli in the water until tender. Add 1 cup of the salsa, garlic powder, and seasoning blend. Remove from the heat; stir in the crumbled tofu, nutritional yeast, and tahini. Coat a square baking dish with ½ cup of the salsa, which will prevent sticking. Divide the spinach and broccoli mixture among the tortillas, and spoon it down the center of each. Roll up the tortillas and place seam-side down in the salsa-lined baking dish. Spoon the remaining 1 ½ cups salsa over the top of the tortillas.

Cover with tinfoil and bake for 25 minutes, or until heated through.

SWEET PEPPER–COCONUT CORN CHOWDER
Recipe Credit: Kim Campbell, *The PlantPure Nation Cookbook*
(Serves 6)

Ingredients

2 leeks, washed well and sliced

3 carrots, diced

3 garlic cloves, minced

1 jalapeño pepper, seeded and minced

2 red bell peppers, seeded and diced

1 cup water

2 cups frozen corn

One 14-oz. can light coconut milk

3 T nutritional yeast flakes

¼ tsp black pepper

1 tsp sea salt

Two 14-oz. cans chickpeas, rinsed and drained

Preparation

In a stockpot over medium-high heat, sauté the leeks, carrots, garlic, jalapeño pepper, and bell peppers in the water until tender. Add the remaining ingredients and simmer for 10 minutes. Scoop out one-third of the mixture and process in a blender until smooth. Add the mixture from the blender back to the pot and simmer for another 10 minutes.

SPLIT PEA SOUP
Recipe Credit: Michael Klunker

(Serves 4-6)

Ingredients

1 medium onion, peeled and chopped into ½ in. pieces

3 cloves garlic, peeled and smashed, chopped fine

1 cup chopped carrots (about 2 medium) - ½ in. pieces

2 medium russet potatoes, washed well and diced into 1 in. pieces

2 large portobello mushrooms, cleaned and diced into 1 in. pieces

1 14.5 oz. can of diced tomatoes

1 ½ cups green split peas, washed and sorted

5 cups mushroom stock (either homemade or from the store - sub with veggie stock if you don't have access to mushroom stock)

2 T low sodium soy sauce

½ tsp garlic powder

1 tsp onion powder

1 tsp Italian seasoning

½ tsp liquid smoke

Instant Pot (Pressure Cooker) preparation

Turn the Instant Pot to the sauté setting. When it has heated up, add the onions, garlic and carrots and saute for about 5 minutes. Add the carrots, potatoes and mushrooms. Continue to saute for another 5 minutes, stirring the whole time. Add the tomatoes and split peas, and stir well. Add the mushroom stock and the remaining spices and liquid smoke. Stir well and bring to a boil. When it has come to a boil, turn off Instant Pot and put the lid on. Make sure knob is set to pressure position, and set the Instant Pot to manual for 18 minutes.

After 18 minutes, do a quick release.

<u>(Stovetop preparation)</u>

Place a large pot with a secure-fitting lid on stove over medium-high heat. Add onions, garlic and carrots. Saute for 10 minutes, until the onions start to become translucent. Add the potatoes, mushrooms, and tomatoes. Stir well and cook for another 5 minutes.

Add the split peas, mushroom stock, all the spices and the liquid smoke. Stir well and allow to come to a simmer. Reduce heat to medium low, and cover tight. Let simmer for about 40 minutes. After 40 minutes, take the lid off and stir well, all the way to the bottom. Check the potatoes and peas. If there is anything not cooked, cover and let cook another 10 minutes. Serve hot.

POWERHOUSE SALAD
By Michael Klunker
(Serves 2-4)

Ingredients
1 lb. fresh Brussels sprouts, trimmed and sliced thin
½ lb. fresh broccoli, trimmed and sliced thin
¼ lb. Tuscan kale (dinosaur kale), washed, massaged and sliced into thin strips
1 15oz. can of great northern beans, drained and rinsed
2 medium carrots, peeled and shredded
½ cup organic (if you can find) raisins
1 large red bell pepper, washed and sliced thin

Preparation
Combine all of the above in a large bowl. Use your hands and mix well. Cover and set in the fridge for a half hour to chill. While it is chilling, prepare dressing.

Dressing Ingredients
½ cup fresh lemon juice
Zest of one lemon
½ block of firm silken tofu
½ cup maple syrup
2 T of white miso
Dash of salt and pepper

Preparation
Combine all the dressing ingredients into a blender and blend until very smooth. You will not need a lot of dressing for the salad, so you can use on other salads or maybe even a baked potato. For best results, let the dressing chill before use

CILANTRO-LIME BREAKFAST POTATOES
By Michael Klunker
(Serves 2-4)

Ingredients
4 medium russet potatoes, washed, cut in half lengthwise, then cut those halves into half and slice into ¼ in. slices
2 cloves garlic, peeled and minced fine
1 tsp salt
1 T low sodium soy sauce
½ tsp pepper (optional)
1 tsp onion powder
¾ cup unseasoned breadcrumbs (I use panko that I put in a blender)
1-2 tsp wasabi powder (or wasabi paste if you have it pre-made)
1 large lime, cut in half
2 T chopped, fresh cilantro

Preparation
Preheat oven to 450° F.
In a large pot, add potatoes, salt and garlic. Add about 6 cups of water, just enough to cover the potatoes by about 1/2 inch. Place on stove and set to medium high. Cover and let come to a soft boil. Remove lid and boil for 10 minutes, or until almost cooked through. Remove from heat and drain. Place back into pot, and add the soy sauce and stir carefully to coat. (Be careful not to break the potatoes) Add the pepper, onion powder, wasabi powder and breadcrumbs, then stir around and coat well, until all the pieces are covered in seasoning and breadcrumbs. ***(If you are using wasabi paste, mix into the soy sauce until blended well, then pour on the potatoes as above)

Place on a baking sheet lined with parchment or a silicone pad. Spread out into one layer. Place in oven and bake for 20-25 minutes, stirring about half way through. For best results, cook until crispy. (Watch them as ovens vary.)

Remove from oven and squeeze the juice from limes all over the potatoes, and serve. Sprinkle with cilantro just before eating.

SPANISH OMELET
By Michael Klunker
(Serves 4-6)

Ingredients
3 medium-sized potatoes (russet or Yukon Gold) peeled, cut in half, and cut into half-moons about ¼ inch thick. Soak for 5 minutes in water. (Keeps them from turning brown.)
1 medium yellow onion, peeled and cut in half. Sliced into half-moons about 1/4 inch thick
½ tsp salt
¼ tsp black pepper (optional)
1 tsp onion powder
1 tsp garlic powder
½ tsp smoked paprika
1 cup water
4 oz. firm tofu (¼ of a brick)
½ tsp baking powder
¾ cup unflavored/unsweetened plant milk
3 T maseca masa flour (corn flour used for tortillas and tamales)
¼ tsp salt

Preparation
In a large, good, nonstick pan, add the onions, potatoes, salt, pepper, onion powder, garlic powder, and smoked paprika. Pour the 1 cup of water over it, and set on the stove over medium heat. Stir around to mix the spices, and cover the pan. Allow to simmer for about 15 minutes, or until the potatoes are cooked.
While they are cooking, make the batter. Add the tofu, baking powder, plant milk, corn flour and salt to a blender and blend until very smooth.

Set aside. When the potatoes are cooked, remove to a colander to drain. Wash the pan out.

Turn the heat to medium low. Place back on the heat, and add the batter. Add the drained potato mixture and press them gently into the batter. Make sure the heat is on medium low, and cover the pan. Walk away. This will take about 15 minutes on the first side. Don't touch it or try to flip it. Just let it do its own thing!

After 15 minutes, use a thin spatula and run around the edges, and slowly around under the omelet. If it starts to tear or seems wet, let it go another 5 minutes and try again.

Once you loosen the omelet, slowly tip the pan and transfer the omelet to a dinner plate. Wipe the pan out and turn the pan onto the plate. Flip the omelet into the pan (I use a hot pad on the bottom of the plate so I don't burn myself) Now, let it cook for another 15-20 minutes.

This time do not cover.

After 15-20 minutes, run your spatula around the edges again, and around the bottom. If it still jiggles, let it go a little longer. Gently remove from pan by tipping it and letting it slide onto a plate.

It will need to set up for about 10 minutes. Do not cover.

This is best served warm, not hot. Cut into wedges and serve with fresh cut tomatoes.

VEG-TRADITIONAL HUNGARIAN GOULASH
By Michael Klunker

(Serves 4-6)

Ingredients

3 large yellow onions, peeled and cut into 1/2 in. cubes

5 cloves garlic, peeled and chopped

3 medium carrots, peeled and cut into 1/2 in. rounds

1 large red bell pepper, washed and seeded, cut into 1/2 in. pieces

1 large green bell pepper, washed and seeded, cut into 1/2 in. pieces

2 large roma tomatoes, washed and cut into 1/2 in. pieces

3 medium yukon gold potatoes, washed and cut into 1/2 in. pieces

1 lb. cremini mushrooms, cleaned and cut in half

3 T Hungarian paprika

1 T smoked paprika

1 bay leaf

1 tsp salt (optional)

½ tsp black pepper

1 T tomato paste

4 cups good veggie stock

2 T corn starch

¼ cup water

Preparation

In a large pot, add the onions and garlic and saute over medium heat. Saute for about 10 minutes, or until they are starting to get translucent. Add the two paprikas and bay leaf and stir well. Cook another minute, then add all the rest of the veggies. Stir them well and cook for 5 minutes more. Add the salt and pepper and add the veggie stock. Stir again well, and allow to come to a simmer over medium heat.

When it comes to a simmer add the tomato paste and stir until it is mixed in, then cover and reduce the heat to low, and walk away.

Cook for 30 minutes.

When it is done cooking, combine the corn starch and ¼ cup of water into a slurry. Turn the heat to medium high, and let the goulash come to a simmer. Add the slurry and stir well. Allow to thicken for 1 minute.

Serve hot, with some plant based sour cream.

You could serve over rice or noodles too.

CREAMY POTATO BROCCOLI SOUP
By Michael Klunker
(Serves 4-6)

Ingredients
1 medium onion, peeled and chopped
3 cloves garlic, peeled and smashed
2 medium russet potatoes, skinned and cubed (approx. 1 in.)
1 medium head of cauliflower, washed and cut into florets.
2 medium parsnips, peeled and cubed (again, 1 inch)
3 cups broccoli florets, washed
½ tsp dry thyme (or 1 tsp fresh, chopped fine)
½ tsp white pepper
4 cups good vegetable stock
2 cups unflavored, non dairy milk.
¼ -½ cup nutritional yeast (you can adjust this if you are not a fan of nutritional yeast)
Optional ingredients:
salt (or salt substitute) to taste
1 tsp browning sauce
½ tsp nutmeg (more if you like)

Preparation
In a large pot, over medium heat, saute the onions and garlic in 2 tablespoons of the stock you are using. You will want to saute for about 8 minutes until the onion starts to soften. If you need to add more stock, do so to prevent sticking. Before you go to the next step, if you are using browning sauce, add that now.
When the onions are nice and soft, start adding the veggies. Start with the potatoes and parsnips. Saute them with the onions for about

5 minutes. Add the rest of the veggies listed, except the broccoli and stir very well.

Add the thyme and the liquid (stock and milk) and give it a good stir. Cover and bring to a simmer over medium heat. Allow to cook for 5 minutes covered. No peeking! After 5 minutes, add the broccoli on top. Cover again and let cook for about 12-15 minutes. After that time, check the veggies and see if they are soft. If not soft, cover and cook for another 5-10 minutes. At this point if you are adding salt, do so.

Take off the heat and with an immersion blender, puree all the veggies. Don't cheat this part, really get in there and make this soup nice and creamy.

After you have achieved a nice consistency, stir in the nutritional yeast, and return to the heat. Keep stirring and cook for another 5 minutes. If the soup is too thick, add more milk or stock to your liking. Also check the seasoning too.

Serve hot and enjoy!!

BERRY BAKED OATMEAL
By Michael Klunker

(Serves 2)

Ingredients
Preheat oven to 375 F.

2 cups cashew milk (or any non-dairy milk)
¼ cup maple syrup
¼ cup date paste
2T chia seeds (you could used ground flax seed also)
1 tsp ground cinnamon
2 tsp vanilla extract (always the real stuff)
2 cups oats (not instant)
2 T chopped walnuts or almonds
⅔ cup frozen or fresh blueberries
1 ⅓ cups quartered frozen or fresh strawberries
⅔ cup fresh or frozen blackberries

Preparation

In a large bowl, combine the first 6 ingredients. Whisk until well blended. Let stand for 10 minutes.

While the liquid is sitting, combine the next 5 ingredients in a 9 in. x 13 in. pan.

After the liquid is ready, whisk one more time and pour over the oat mixture.

Make sure that the liquid is evenly distributed. Tilting the pan around and then holding it up to look under it to make sure the liquid had gone to the bottom helps.

Place in the oven and bake for 35-40 minutes. You want the top to be a deep, rich brown.

Remove from oven, and let sit uncovered for 10 minutes. This part is important. (Much easier to remove)

Serve hot or room temp. Add extra fresh berries on the side if you would like.

SPICY SWEET POTATO TACOS
By Michael Klunker
(Serves 2-4)

Ingredients
1 medium sweet potato, peeled and sliced into "fry" sized slices
1 medium yellow onion, peeled, cut in half and cut into half moon slices.
(about ¼-inch thick)
8-10 medium mushrooms, cleaned and sliced into thin slices
½ a red bell pepper, washed and cut into ½-in. pieces
½ cup frozen corn
1 tsp onion powder
1 tsp garlic powder
½ tsp salt
½ tsp pepper
½ tsp chipotle powder
½ tsp cumin

Preparation
In a large, nonstick pan, add the sweet potatoes, and about 1/4 cup water. Cover with a lid and set on medium-high heat. Steam for about 5 minutes, or until almost tender. Remove lid and add all the other veggies. Cook until the onions are translucent and everything is soft. Add the spices and mix well (but carefully, so you don't break down the sweet potatoes)
After everything is cooked well, and sweet potatoes are soft, remove from heat.
Scoop mix into taco shells. Top with salsa, avocado, cilantro, or any favorite taco toppings.

CURRY-DIJON QUINOA SALAD

Recipe Credit: Katie Mae, PlantBasedKatie.com
(Serves 4)

Ingredients
3½ cups cooked quinoa (about 1 cup dry)
1 cup water
¼ - ½ cup cashews
1½ T stone-ground or Dijon mustard
1½ T apple cider vinegar
1½ T curry powder
½ T garlic granules
1 date, pitted (or 4 oz. apple)
1 apple (about 6 oz.)
¼ cup red onion, diced (about 3 oz.)
3 cups spinach, diced (about 3 oz.)
½ lemon, juiced

Preparation
In a blender, add water, cashews, Dijon, apple cider vinegar, curry powder, garlic granules and date. Blend until smooth and creamy.
In a large bowl add the apple, onion, spinach, and cooked quinoa. Gently fold the curry sauce it into the dry ingredients.
Squeeze lemon over top the salad and gently mix the salad once more. Serve at room temp or chill in the fridge and enjoy later.

AFRICAN YAM STEW

Recipe Credit: Katie Mae, PlantBasedKatie.com

(Serves 6-8)

Ingredients

1 onion, chopped

1-2 T jalapeno pepper, minced

1 T ginger, ground

1 T garlic granules

2 tsp cumin, ground

2 tsp coriander, ground

¼ tsp crushed red pepper

6 yams, peeled and chopped

2 cups water

24 oz. tomatoes, chopped

1½ cups (15 oz.) garbanzo beans, (1 can, drained and rinsed)

1½ cups (15 oz.) black eyed peas, (1 can, drained and rinsed)

½ cup almond or peanut butter, unsweetened

1½ cups organic corn

1 bunch collards or kale, chopped

Preparation

In a large pot over medium heat, add onion and pepper, but no oil. Cover with lid to keep the moisture released from the veggies in the pan. Stir frequently to prevent the veggies from sticking. Add ginger, garlic, cumin, coriander and red pepper. Cook for a couple more minutes, continuing to stir.

Add yams, water, tomatoes, beans and nut butter. Bring to a boil, reduce heat and simmer for 20 minutes.

Stir in corn and collards and cook for about 10 more minutes, until yams and greens are tender. To make this dish a little lighter, serve over raw leafy greens. For extra heartiness, serve over brown rice or other whole grain.

BBQ BEANS AND GREENS

Recipe Credit: Katie Mae, PlantBasedKatie.com

(Serves 4-6)

Beans and Greens Ingredients

1 small yellow onion, diced

1½ bunches of kale, de-stemmed chopped (any type)

1½ cup cooked cannellini beans (1 can, no salt-added, rinsed)

1½ cup cooked pinto beans (1 can, no salt-added, rinsed)

BBQ Sauce Ingredients

¾ cup warm water

5 dates, pitted

6 oz. can of tomato paste

8 oz. canned pineapple with juice (no sugar added)

2 T apple cider vinegar

2 T stone ground mustard

1 T smoked paprika

1 T garlic granules (or powder)

1 T chili powder

½ T onion flakes (or powder)

Preparation

In a food processor or blender, combine BBQ sauce ingredients. Blend to even consistency and set aside.

In a large saucepan over medium heat, place onions and cook with lid on, stirring occasionally, for about 5 minutes until onions are translucent. With a lid on pan the water that sweats out from onions is kept in pan, and thus there is no need to start with water or oil.

Add the beans and chopped kale to the onions. Cook for a few minutes, stirring occasionally. If mixture is too dry, add less than ¼ cup of water. Add the BBQ sauce to the beans and greens. Gently toss mixture so everything is covered with sauce. Cook on low for 5-10 minutes to incorporate the flavors, then serve.

SPICY TEMPEH STIR FRY

Recipe Credit: Katie Mae, PlantBasedKatie.com
(Serves 2)

Ingredients
1 red onion, sliced
1 bell pepper, sliced
2 cups sugar snap peas
1 T cumin, ground
½–1 T chili powder
8 oz. plain tempeh, sliced
1 lime, juiced
¼ cup cilantro, diced
2 T pumpkin seeds (raw or toasted)

Preparation
Add vegetables and spices to a sauté pan over medium-high heat and cover with a lid. Some browning is desirable as it adds flavor, but stir often so the veggies don't burn. Let the spices toast for a few minutes.
Then add the tempeh and lime juice. Keep the pan covered but continue to stir frequently. If the pan becomes too dry and veggies are starting to stick, then add a little water or vegetable broth as needed.
After the tempeh has fully cooked, about 7-8 minutes, transfer to a serving bowl or individual bowls. Sprinkle with fresh cilantro and pumpkin seeds.

FAVORITE WEBSITES

www.wholefoodplantbased.info - my blog site.

www.forksoverknives.com - the film that started it all!

www.nutritionfacts.org - great videos from Dr. Michael Greger.

www.drmcdougall.com - be sure to visit the forums section, the central gathering place for Whole-Food Plant-Based living.

www.dresselstyn.com - Dr. Caldwell Esselstyn.

www.nutritionstudies.org - the T. Colin Campbell Center for Nutrition Studies – home of the certificate program in conjuction with eCornell (highly recommended!)

www.pcrm.org - Physicians Committee for Responsible Medicine – great legislative work and research.

www.happycow.net - the resource for finding vegan and vegetarian restaurants worldwide.

www.happyherbivore.com - great source of recipes from Lindsay Nixon, the "Happy Herbivore".

www.eatunprocessed.com - Chef AJ – wonderful recipes and videos.

www.plantpurenation.com - grassroots education and action-oriented network.

www.engine2diet.com - Rip Esselstyn's twist on the Whole-Food Plant-Based diet (Dr. Esselstyn's son).

www.vegsource.com - great source of articles, links and news

www.richroll.com - world class ultra-athlete with a remarkable story to tell.

www.brendadavisrd.com - one of the world's authorities on nutrition.

www.comfortablyunaware.com - Dr. Richard Oppenlander – author of two fabulous books on the environment and sustainability. Do not miss these books!

www.healthpromoting.com - TrueNorth Health Center, led by Dr. Alan Goldhamer. Fascinating treatment for an array of chronic health problems at their center in Santa Rosa.

FAVORITE BOOKS & FILMS

www.wfpbbooks.com - shop the bookstore I've put together to browse through more than 40 books and 5 films I have enjoyed.

ENDNOTES

Chapter Two

1. *The whole premise of the diet is torn to shreds Ted Talk given by Christina Warinner*: http://tedxtalks.ted.com/video/Debunking-the-Paleo-Diet-Christ

2. *Ibid.*

3. *"As to the grain/legume consumption itself, it still begs the questions of what is really healthy to eat, particularly as a preponderanceofcalories?"* http://robbwolf.com/2013/04/04/debunking-paleo-diet-wolfs-eye-view

4. *usually estimated at no more than thirty-five* http://wholehealthsource.blogspot.com/2008/08/life-expectancy-and-growth-of.html

5. *with a not terribly enviable life expectancy in the mid-sixties* http://www.statcan.gc.ca/daily-quotidien/080123/dq080123d-eng.htm

6. *...Nutrition factors of high protein, high nitrogen, high phosphorus, and low calcium intakes may be implicated."* Mazess RB, Mather W. "Bone mineral content of North Alaskan Eskimos." The American Journal of Clinical Nutrition 1974;27:916-25.

7. *A 1935 study of fat vs. carbohydrate consumption in various cultures showed that as carbohydrate intake increases and fat intake decreases, mortality associated with diabetes plummets by about 86%.* Himsworth H.P. "Diet and the incidence of diabetes mellitus." Clin Sci. 2 (1935): 117-148. As cited by Campbell, T. Colin, *The China Study*, (Dallas, BenBella Books, 2006), p.149

8. *"nutrients from animal-based foods increased tumor development while nutrients from plant-based foods decreased tumor development."* Campbell, T. Colin, *The China Study*, p.66

9. *Vegans had the lowest risk of heart disease and stroke due to lower blood pressure.* Appleby, P.N. et al, "Hypertension and blood pressure among meat eaters, fish eaters, vegetarians, and vegans in EPIC-Oxford," Public Health Nutr, 2002 Oct; 5:645-54.

10. *A 1996 study of more than 50,000 male health professionals demonstrated that those who ate the most fiber had a reduced risk of coronary heart disease.* Rimm, Eric, "Vegetable, fruit, and cereal intake and risk of coronary heart disease among men," Journal of the American Medical Association, 1996, Feb.14 (275:447).

11. *Another study, this one of over 25,000 Seventh-Day Adventists in California, found that daily meat-eaters had a three times greater likelihood of dying from heart disease than those who did not eat meat.* Snowdon, D.A. et al, "Meat consumption and fatal ischemic heart disease," Prev Med, Sep 1984; 13(5):490-500

12. Dr. Milton Mills...makes perhaps the most clear and definitive analysis of the diet we humans were designed to eat in his essay, "The Comparative Anatomy of Eating." http://www.adaptt.org/Mills%20The%20Comparative%20Anatomy%20of%20Eating1.pdf

13. *"...we have something much more powerful: high intelligence, which allowed humans to become the most efficient hunters, and the dominant mammalian species, on the planet."* http://www.beyondveg.com/billings-t/comp-anat/comp-anat-6a.shtml

Chapter Three

1. *"…This rapid absorption tends to injure the liver, glycates protein and injures the endothelial cells."* (http://www.dresselstyn.com/site/faq/)

2. McDougall, John, *The Starch Solution* (N.Y., N.Y, Rodale Books, 2012) p.8

3. McDougall, Ibid., p.13

4. *"…you're basking that cauldron of inflammation with nature's most powerful anti-oxidants all day long."* https://www.youtube.com/watch?v=-7mYblX4ugE

5. *Population studies have demonstrated repeatedly that people who eat five servings or more of fruits and vegetables have about half the risk of developing many types of cancer.* Boivin, Dominique et al, "Antiproliferative and antioxidant activities of common vegetables: A comparative study," Food Chemistry 112 (2009) 374-380

6. *And yet only 14% of Americans eat the recommended five servings per day of fruits (2 fruits) and vegetables (3 vegetables).* http://usato-day30.usatoday.com/news/health/2009-09-29-fruits-veggies-high-school-kids_N.htm

7. *According to the CDC, the average American actually eats 1.1 fruits per day and 1.6 vegetables per day.* http://www.cdc.gov/nutrition/downloads/State-Indicator-Report-Fruits-Vegetables-2013.pdf

8. *…and this is including canned fruits and vegetables and French fries.* http://www.pbhfoundation.org/pdfs/about/res/pbh_res/State_of_the_Plate_2015_WEB_Bookmarked.pdf

9. ... individuals who eat five servings or more of fruits and vegetables daily have approximately half the risk of developing a wide variety of cancer types, particularly those of the gastrointestinal tract." Boivin, Dominique et al, op cit.

10. *In the first decade of this century, a study was conducted in Thessaly, Greece, of 120 people who suffer from COPD...* E. Keranis et al, "Impact of dietary shift to higher-antioxidant foods in COPD: a randomised trial" European Respiratory Journal, October 1, 2010 vol. 36 no. 4 774-780

11. *...the percentage of five year survival after being diagnosed with esophageal cancer is 38% for localized cancer to the esophagus (and much less if the cancer has already spread beyond the esophagus).* http://www.webmd.com/digestive-disorders/esophageal-cancer?page=3#1

12. *At the end of six months, the treatment reversed the lesions of 29 of those 36 patients.* Chen, T. et al "Randomized phase II trial of lyophilized strawberries in patients with dysplastic precancerous lesions of the esophagus." Cancer Prev Res (Phila). 2012 Jan;5(1):41-50

13. *...the capacity to disrupt tumor blood supply has been found in specific phytochemicals present in tea, spices, fruit, and beans.* Reuben, Sharon C. et al, "Modulation of angiogenesis by dietary phytoconstituents in the prevention and intervention of breast cancer." Mol Nutr Food Res. 2012 Jan;56(1):14-29.

14. *As little as five button mushrooms per day may do the trick to protect women from breast cancer.* "White Button Mushroom Phytochmeicals Inhibit Aromatase Activity and Breast Cancer Cell

Proliferation" Grube, Baiba J. et al, J. Nutr. Dec. 1, 2001, vol 131, no 12, 3288-3293

15. *Buettner recommends eating a cup of beans per day.* Buettner, Dan, The Blue Zones Solution: Eating and Living Like the World's Healthiest People (National Geographic, 2015, p?)

16. *In fact, the foods that excel in this regard are collard greens, kale, mustard greens, broccoli, and cabbage—and to get their full bile-acid-binding effect, steam them.* Kahlon, T.S. et al, "Steam cooking significantly improves in vitro bile acid binding of collard greens, kale, mustard greens, broccoli, green bell pepper, and cabbage." Nutr Res. 2008 Jun;28(6):351-7.

17. *The champions are Swiss chard, basil, beet greens, spring greens, butter lettuce, arugula, cilantro, and rhubarb.* Webb, AJ et al, "Acute blood pressure lowering, vasoprotective, and antiplatelet properties of dietary nitrate via bioconversion to nitrite," Hypertension. 2008 Mar;51(3):784-90.

Chapter Four

1. *"...The major storyline in the film traces the personal journeys of a pair of pioneering yet under-appreciated researchers, Dr. T. Colin Campbell and Dr. Caldwell Esselstyn."* http://www.forksoverknives.com/synopsis/

2. *After losing the weight, my story was told in such media outlets as CNN and The Globe, as well as on Dr. McDougall's website.* http://foodasmedicine.info/press-kit/

3. *"...livestock and their byproducts actually account for at least (emphasis theirs)...51% of annual worldwide GHG (greenhouse gas) emissions."* [p.11] *"26% of land worldwide is dedicated to grazing livestock,*

and one-third of arable land is used to grow feed." [p.13] Robert Goodland and Jeff Anhang https://cgspace.cgiar.org/bitstream/handle/10568/10601/IssueBrief3.pdf

4. *As of 2012, the CDC reports that half of all adults have one or more chronic condition. One in four has two or more chronic conditions. In 2010, 7 of the top 10 causes of death in this country were chronic, preventable diseases. Here's the real kicker: 84% of all health care spending in 2006 was spent on the 50% of our population who have one or more chronic conditions that can be prevented or controlled with diet. The total cost of heart disease and stroke in 2010 was 315 billion dollars. On diabetes? 245 billion. And medical costs linked to obesity were 128 billion dollars in 2003.* http://www.cdc.gov/chronicdisease/overview

Acknowledgements

Special thanks go to my coauthor, Glen Merzer, whom I have enjoyed getting to know over the past couple years, and with whom I had a great time putting this book together. I am honored that he agreed to take this project on.

Thanks to our wonderful editor Nicole Schlosser, who worked at odd hours to help us get to press on time.

Thanks to a new friend, Shannon Gotto, who not only designed the "Food is My Healthcare" T-shirt I'm wearing on the front cover (yours is available at ecovegangal.com, by the way), but also did extensive design work for the production of this book, as well as many Remedy Food Project designs that are in the works.

Thank you to all of our contributing recipe authors. It's been an embarrassment of riches to have so many delicious recipes made available to us to share with you.

Thank you to the pioneers of plant-based nutrition who helped to change my life and so many lives worldwide. I sincerely hope that my generation and those who follow will be able to take the lessons they have shared and continue to educate the masses about proper human nutrition – for human health, for the environment, for animal welfare and for our economy.

To my friends and family, thank you for your support during my journey, and for being open-minded and asking questions about this "radical" lifestyle.

To my parents, who gave me the moral compass and ethics that have led me to this unexpected fork in the road, many thanks.

Lastly, thank you to my partner in life, Claire, who has not only accompanied me on this plant-based journey, but has supported this and every effort I have undertaken since we first met in high school. I think we make a pretty good team!

About the Authors

Benji Kurtz is a self-described serial entrepreneur who changed to a plant-based lifestyle in 2013 and hasn't looked back. He is the founder and Executive Director of Remedy Food Project, a Georgia-based non-profit (www.remedyfood.org). Kurtz was educated at Emory University and holds a certificate in Plant-Based Nutrition from eCornell & The T. Colin Campbell Center for Nutrition Studies. Kurtz and his wife Claire reside in Atlanta.

Glen Merzer is a playwright, screenwriter, and author. Glen's first novel is *Off the Reservation*, the story of a vegan congressman's quest for the presidency. Merzer is also the co-author of *Mad Cowboy* and *No More Bull!*, with Howard Lyman; *Better Than Vegan*, with Chef Del Sroufe; *Unprocessed*, with Chef AJ; and *Food Over Medicine*, with Pam Popper.